Black Culture and Mental Health

Robin R. Lomax

ACKNOWLEDGEMENTS

Through this program, I have met amazing professors, peers, colleagues, and friends who encouraged me along the way! Dr. Longnecker, thank you for pushing me beyond my limits! You helped me to see that a challenge only remains a challenge if you give up!

To my mentor, Mr. Chris Ramsey, thank you for believing in me and giving me those needed pep-talks throughout this journey. I will continue to be the change and follow the path God has written for me. Rest in Power!

To my friends, I am forever grateful for your patience, your support, your prayers, your words of encouragement, and your love. It is a blessing to have people in your corner who truly believe in you and want to see you win!

This dissertation study was completed to give those within my community a voice and to advocate on their behalf. Black women and men, there are safe spaces such as therapy for you to heal! To the Black mental health professionals, thank you for your service and advocacy! Your knowledge and impeccable work speak volumes as we continue to raise awareness of mental health within our communities!

DEDICATION

This dissertation is dedicated to my mother, Marcie, my great-grandmother, Louise Davis, and my family for their words of encouragement, prayers, love, and support during my doctoral journey. Mom, I could not have traveled along this journey without you. Thank you for being my prayer partner, for holding me accountable, and for supporting me. I love you more than words can express. Bigmama, you are no longer here on Earth with us, but your spirit lives on and kept me going throughout this journey. I know in moments of doubt, you were pulling me through. To my family, thank you for your continuous support, your prayers, and love; for that I am forever grateful!

ABSTRACT

The purpose of this research study was to explore the careers of Black/African American women and men in the mental health field and to examine the experiences of the Black/African American culture to begin breaking the cycle of the underutilization of therapeutic services for mental health. This study captured the experiences and perspectives of the Black/African American community from two separate groups in which created a gateway to increase awareness of mental health.

TABLE OF CONTENTS

Chapter	Page
I. INTRODUCTION	1
Statement of the Problem	2
Rationale	6
Research Questions or Hypotheses	13
Description of Terms	14
Contribution of the Study	15
Process to Accomplish	18
Conclusion	29
II. REVIEW OF THE LITERATURE	30
Introduction	30
Historical Overview	31
Global Mental Health	34
Mental Illness Within the Culture	36
Stakeholders	39
The Black Family: The Role of Support	42
Religion and the Role it Plays within the Black Culture	44
Barriers Seeking Mental Health	46
Cultural Competency and Cultural Intelligence	50
Phenomenological Theory	53

	Continuous Oppression Impacting Mental Health..54
	Counselors as Transformation Leaders within the Community............................56
	Conclusion 57
III.	METHODOLOGY 59
	Introduction..59
	Research Design...60
	Participants...60
	Data Collection 62
	Analytical Methods..66
	Conclusion..69
IV.	FINDINGS AND CONCLUSIONS 70

Chapter	Page
Introduction	70
Findings	71
Summary of the Findings	83
Limitations	84
Implications and Recommendations	86
Conclusion	88

LIST OF FIGURES

Figure   Page

1. Highlighted Themes During Individual Interviews 71

2. Curated Themes During Individual Interviews and Focus Group…………...78

CHAPTER I

INTRODUCTION

The history of mental illness for black people in America stretches all the way back 400 years, 15 million people, and an ocean that holds the stories - Nissen

In recent studies, Black/African American women and men were not seeking therapy or mental health services due to underrepresentation of licensed Black/African American therapists, social workers, or mental health professionals (Taylor & Kuo, 2018). In 2013, Dr. Jeff R. Gardere, an African American psychologist, reported that Black/African Americans would seek mental health services if there were more racial-ethnic clinicians (Smith, 2015). He expressed that it could help eliminate the mistrust that Black/African Americans may feel when seeking therapy services from those not of their race. The SAMHSA workforce report noted that within the White/Non-Hispanic community, 55.8% were mental/behavioral health professionals and 27.9% of Black/African Americans were mental/behavioral health professionals. It was estimated that within those racial and ethnic minorities that 19.2% were psychiatrists, 17.5% were social workers, 10.3% were counselors, 7.8% were marriage and family therapists, and 5.1% were psychologists (Smith, 2015).

The Black/African American culture agrees that mental health services are needed but are still on the fence about seeking and receiving services (Ward et al., 2013). The National Alliance on Mental Illness (NAMI) African American Community Mental Health Fact Sheet reported that the representation of Black/African American mental health professionals were very low with only 2% being psychiatrists, 2% being psychologists, and 4% being social workers in the United States (Smith, 2015). It is a necessity to have more representation of Black/African American women and men in the field of behavioral/mental health to impede the obstacles of Black/African Americans gaining access to psychotherapy and mental health services (Taylor & Kuo, 2018). Research suggests that if clients see their culture reflected in psychologists, therapists, and mental health professionals, the culture will buy into mental health services (Ward et al., 2013). In the past, the Black/African American culture looked at therapeutic services as taboo and ineffective due to religious reasoning, leading to the underutilization of mental health services in the community (Hatcher, King, Barnett, & Burler, 2016).

Statement of the Problem

The purpose of this research was to explore the careers of Black/African American women and men in the mental health field and to examine the experiences of the Black/African American culture to begin breaking the cycle of not receiving or a lack of therapeutic services for mental health. This study explored barriers of potential Black/African American clients receiving mental health services, challenges that mental health professionals face when working with clients of their culture, what practices led to engagement of services, and the mental health professionals have reached positive outcomes with the Black/African American clients they see. While learning how mental health has affected the Black/African American culture, the readers gain a better understanding of how important it is for there to be a broader representation of Black/African American mental health professionals as well as how vital it is to increase educational awareness of mental health services/ resources within the communities they serve

Mental health has been categorized as a form of health disparity within the Black/African American culture, but mental health services are underutilized due to barriers and lack of access to culturally competent providers (Hatcher et al., 2016). Mental health is an issue that several have been faced with, and some have sought out treatment, yet others have not due to fear of being judged, misdiagnosed, the stigma behind the diagnosis, and lack of insurance to cover the therapeutic expenses (Kohn-Wood & Hooper, 2014).

The cultural stressors and barriers towards seeking mental health within the African American culture have led to negative imagery of therapeutic and behavioral health services (Smith, 2015). The negativity behind seeking and receiving mental health services has a lot to do with the racism and fear that clinicians of the opposite race would project their prejudices onto them due to cultural differences (Knifton, 2012). Black/African American women and men entering the field can change the narrative and motivate those within the culture to seek psychological services within the community by being the mental health advocates one trusts (Taylor & Kuo, 2018).

A significant component of behavior/mental health is understanding cultural competency and releasing some of the strain faced when treating Black/African American clients (Smith, 2015). Therapists have faced early withdrawal of clients from therapy due to lack of social support or lack of understanding what psychotherapy is as far as treatment is concerned (Williams, 2011). By being aware of one's own culture and values and being knowledgeable of the clients they serve, clinicians began to research terminology that would better help them grasp the skepticism towards therapy, such as stigma (Smith, 2015). "Stigmatization may affect not just people with mental health difficulties, but also, by association, their families" (Tew et al., 2011, p.7). It has been noted that people diagnosed with mental illness are looked at differently, and because of the stereotyping or stigma, one may not be able to gain employment or afford other opportunities that others without mental health issues would be able to gain (Tew et al., 2011). There is an urgent need to implement procedures to improve treatment amongst the Black/African American culture (Williams, 2011). Mental health providers, which consist of counselors, social workers, psychologists, and psychiatrists, are expected to provide proper treatment regardless of race or ethnicities to eradicate the untreated mental health illness in their communities (Kohn-Wood & Hooper, 2014).

While cultural competency is a significant component of gaining buy-in from the Black/African American community to seek and receive mental health services, there are other practices that potential clients would like to see to broaden their mindsets regarding mental health services (Hatcher et al., 2016). Those practices consist of having more representation of Black/African American men and women as therapists in the mental health field and being better informed and trained to implement theories and practices that align with the client's religion and spirituality (Hatcher et al., 2016). Seeking mental health services is growing within the culture, but some potential clients feel uneasy seeking or receiving mental health services (Williams, 2011). Older generations instilled relying on the spiritual realm to take care of their problems and help heal the body, whether physically or mentally, and it continues to be a significant source for Black/African American culture (Hatcher et al., 2016). Therefore, clinicians should gain an understanding of how religion and spirituality play a role in the client's overall well-being to create a client-centered treatment plan to obtain success with the client during therapy (Avent, Cashwell, & Brown-Jeffy, 2015).

Mental health professionals advocate, influence, impact, and serve those in need in their communities. Black/African American Therapists have implemented practices to serve clients in their communities to see progress in their mental health. One way to approach better treatment regarding race and culture was to modify the treatment, such as the delivery of the evidence-based treatment to honor the cultural beliefs and behaviors of the Black/African American population (Ward & Brown, 2015). Researchers have noted that within Black/African American communities, stigma, racism, and religious/spiritual beliefs have contributed to reduced access to mental health services (Taylor & Kuo, 2018; Smith, 2015). However, by incorporating the Afrocentric perspective into mental health practice when seeing Black/African American clients, therapists have experienced growth with their clients over time (Hatcher et al., 2016). Researchers believe that using the Eurocentric theory demeans and diminishes the culture of Black/African Americans, which is not effective and unethical (Hatcher et al., 2016). Eurocentrism is the theory of incorporating the White European race's values, traditions, and cultural norms into other races and ethnicities despite the difference in racial and cultural norms (Awosan, Sandberg, & Hall, 2011).

Hatcher et al., (2016) noted in their literature that:

> The African-centered philosophy, a system based on holistic values and ways of living, counters the pathological approach that many mainstream workers chose to utilize when dealing with African Americans and other groups of color and insists

on practice that honors cultural uniqueness, personal strengths, and community development. (Hatcher et al., 2016, p. 5)

This will allow self-empowerment to take place during face-to-face clinical sessions with clients and restore hope. To further explore what produces success amongst Black/African American clients in engagement of services, mental health professionals have implemented the client's own environment into their healing process. Those within the social work field have implemented working with the client's overall social supports, which includes their environmental factors to develop appropriate treatment plans that could lead to success with their client (Hatcher et al., 2016).

Rationale

Mental illness is common in all races and ethnicities, but it can be a heavier stressor for some cultures than others. According to the U.S. Census Bureau, in 2007, Black/African Americans accounted for 12% of the population but accounted for 18.7% of those affected by mental illness (Ward et al., 2013). It was reported that the underutilization of mental health services was due to mistrust of the provider, non-relational matches of therapists or providers, lack of care or access to care, and financial barriers (Masuda, Anderson, & Edmonds, 2012).

In the past, therapy was not a practice implemented with the Black/African American culture, but recent studies to examine Black/African American beliefs about mental illness and attitudes toward seeking mental health services have shown mixed results. In the past and even now, Black/African Americans feel that being labeled as having mental health issues or seeking mental health services is very stigmatizing (Ward et al., 2013). "Stigma may be defined as a process involving labeling, separation, stereotype awareness, stereotype endorsement, prejudice, and discrimination in a context in which social, economic, or political power is exercised to the detriment of members of a social group" (Clement et al., 2015, p. 11). Furthermore, mental health stigma is described as discrimination against people with mental disorders (Masuda et al., 2012). Due to the inhumane history of Black/African Americans fight through the oppression of slavery and race-based trauma, being discriminated against, and looked down upon has caused delayed responses to significant health disparities within their culture, one being mental health (Williams et al., 2014).

Following the stigma, another barrier is the mistrust of mental health professionals for fear of being misdiagnosed. According to Schwartz and Blankenship (2014), "Assigning a mental disorder diagnosis primarily influenced by personal perceptions of or stereotypes about consumers' ethnicity or culture risks inadvertently harming consumers psychologically or socially through misdiagnosis" (Introduction section, para. 1). A misdiagnosis can be described as giving a client a diagnosis when no symptoms or signs are present or a diagnosis due to similar symptoms as another condition (Schwartz & Blankenship, 2014).

While stigma, mistrust, and being misdiagnosed have been challenges to Black/African Americans seeking mental health services, the financial burden of mental health treatment is a barrier that affects everyone. Black/African Americans are greatly affected due to lack of insurance, lack of employment or reduced employment opportunities, high insurance rates, or not to cover services with the insurance offered (Williams, 2011; Walker, Cummings, Hockenberry, & Druss, 2015). According to Ward and Besson (2012), four visits with a mental health clinician are adequate mental health care (Ward & Besson, 2012). Within the U.S. population, it is estimated that 20% of people with mental disorders do not have insurance (Walker et al., 2015). Although some health care organizations cannot slight the cost, other individual practices and treatment centers can help clients by providing low-cost treatment options. Some private practices do not take insurance and allow clients to pay or have a sliding fee scale (Williams, 2011).

Researchers have found that Black/African American therapists have experienced challenges while working with Black/African American clients due to mistrust, stigma, lack of knowledge of psychotherapy, and early withdrawal from the therapeutic process. Psychologist Monnica T Williams, Ph.D. completed a study in 2011 and found that Black/African Americans seeking treatment felt it would reflect on their families, such as not handling internal conflict and lacking education on what mental illness is and how to seek treatment (Williams, 2011). Clients' concerns reduce the clinician's ability to provide value to the needs of the clients (Hatcher et al., 2016). "Mental health and other medical practitioners may perpetuate poor health outcomes through failure to assess historical perspectives, potentially influencing patient mistrust of healthcare" (Williams et al., 2014, pg.106). Black/African Americans will not see treatment progress when appropriate assessments and treatment plans are not developed. The negative connotation of psychotherapy and the mistrust of clinicians will also prohibit treatment progress, seeing as some clients may not fully participate or engage in therapy (Williams et al., 2014).

When discussing the barriers for Black/African American clients, a significant component is a stigma behind mental illness. Black/African American therapists are challenged to break that stigma by raising awareness of mental health and treating mental health illnesses. Due to African Americans' lack of knowledge, it can be difficult for African American therapists to get buy-in from clients (William, 2011).

Fear is a significant component of Black/African Americans not seeking therapy. The fear derived from past or recent experiences of working with psychologists who used the cultural behavior of their clients to stereotype or misjudge the client (Kohn-Wood & Hooper, 2014). Black/African Americans felt as though those in the mental health professionals were not culturally sensitive to their needs, which formed a negative perspective around being diagnosed (Kohn-Wood & Hooper, 2014). There is a greater need, more so of an obligation, for clinicians to be culturally competent and sensitive to the needs of their clients (Schwartz & Blankenship, 2014). The only way to receive proper treatment is to be seen by a clinician and be screened for a proper diagnosis. The fear has kept many Black/African Americans from receiving the help they need in which the result can lead to the longevity of the mental illness if there is one. Williams noted that psychotherapy works only if the clinician and client are on the same team. There must be a mutual understanding between both the client and clinician, respect from both parties, and that the clinician must continue to be culturally competent to address the client's needs (Williams, 2011).

Furthermore, the skepticism of mental health services leads to therapists losing clients before psychotherapy begins. It is noted that every therapist has experienced a client ending the therapeutic process early (Williams, 2011). Previous research noted that 40%-60% drop out of psychotherapy after their first session (Owen, Imel, Adelson, & Rodolfa, 2012). Furthermore, it was reported that Black/African Americans drop out of psychotherapy and rarely revisit it despite the benefits therapy has to offer (Williams et al., 2014). The term dropping out of therapy sounds negative, but it is the reality of what happens within the therapeutic process. Again, lack of awareness and education and the stigma attached to mental health or mental illness can reduce the engagement of mental health (Williams, 2011). Clinicians define dropping out of therapeutic services as a failure to complete the treatment plan, along with the number of therapeutic sessions a client may need to see progress (Owen et al., 2012). It is reported that the client's diagnosis, therapist-to-client match, and misunderstanding of diagnosis and treatment leads to clients dropping out (Owen et al., 2012). According to Williams (2011), clinicians have the responsibility of explaining the process.

When discussing the idea of breaking barriers, knowledge, and advocacy to raise awareness regarding mental health are necessary for the Black/African American community. Communication and positive experiences with clinicians and clients will produce positive outcomes and progress with African Americans engaging in mental health services (Mulvaney-Day et al., 2011). It was reported that Black/African Americans are not as engaged in psychotherapy and mental health services due to their relational preference of receiving treatment from another Black/African American within the profession. For Black/African Americans to engage in therapy, the clinicians need to understand their history, reluctance and help them work through those issues to move forward with the therapeutic process (Mulvaney-Day et al., 2011).

Potential clients would engage more in psychotherapy if more representations of Black/African Americans in the mental health field. This would gain buy-in from the Black/African American community. The National Alliance reported on Mental Illness

(2004) that In the United States, only 2% of African Americans are psychologists (Beasley, Keino-Miller, & Cokley, 2015). "Black men earned 1% of all doctoral degrees awarded in psychology, whereas Black women represented 5% of all newly minted psychologists (Beasley et al., 2015, p.705). This is a critical issue within the community when raising awareness of mental health issues and seeking mental health services. The community at large prefers relational preference. In an interview with Black/African American community members, it was discussed that Black/African Americans prefer working with Black/African American psychologists due to cultural understanding (Beasley et al., 2015). Potential Black/African American clients feel judged and are not as eager to disclose problems when feeling inferior to the person gaining their personal information. This could cause unwanted conflict and, more so more ill feelings towards seeking mental health. According to Williams (2011), some African Americans feel that White people developed psychotherapy for White people. Therefore, if more Black/African American men and women enter the field as clinicians, more Black/African Americans would be inclined to seek mental health services (Beasley et al., 2015). It is suggested that increasing more Black/African American men and women as clinicians could create a platform for those within the Black/African American community to feel safe and secure with expressing themselves, especially for black/African American boys and men (Beasley et al., 2015).

  The environmental factors that Black/African American males experience as a little boy to an adult can lead to depression, substance use and substance abuse, anxiety, anger issues, posttraumatic stress disorder, and other forms of mental health issues. There is a safe and secure feeling when a client can talk about their mental health with a clinician they can connect with regarding race and culture. "Despite gender norms that may limit sharing with other men, Black men also receive unique messages about viewing other Black men as their brothers who may understand the experiential reality of living as a Black man in a racially oppressive society" (Beasley et al., 2015, p. 707). As more Black/African Americans are represented in this field, it creates an empowerment tool amongst the Black/African American community. Black/African American psychologists and therapists can provide their clients with tools, resources to empower them to take charge of their mental health.

When the community can see people in the profession who look like them and have a connection or commonality in place, often, it releases the anxiety, fears, and negative connotation of what mental health sounds like to them. According to Williams (2011), Black/African Americans are represented in the mental health field as master's level clinicians, social workers, professional counselors, and family and marriage therapists.

"Professional psychologists are equipped to serve as clinicians, researchers, teachers, consultants, clinical supervisors, and administrators as well as psychological, educational, and personality test administrators in a variety of settings, including academic, forensic, and community sites" (Beasley et al., 2015, p.705). Being equipped in this manner means that psychologists have had to research different ideologies, theories, and practices to engage the Black/African American community in psychotherapy (Hatcher et al., 2016). Regarding seeing success with Black/African Americans in mental health services, researchers have maintained that utilizing

Eurocentric theories as a sole perspective to explain the cultural behaviors of Black/African Americans is ineffective and unethical.

Due to the history of African Americans' fear of mistrust of therapeutic services for fear of being misdiagnosed and judged, it was best to find a cultural approach that would help heal instead of hinder growth. As mentioned before, using the African-centered philosophy approach speaks more to one's cultural and personal strengths, which leads to the empowerment of self. According to Hatcher et al., 2016, The Afrocentric theory was rooted in the principles of Kwanzaa, which are: Umoja (Unity), Kujichagulia (Self- determination), Ujima (Collective work and responsibility), Ujamaa (Cooperative economics), Nia (Purpose), Kuumba (Creativity), and Imani (Faith) (Hatcher et al., 2016). Researchers have noted that not every Black/African American celebrates Kwanzaa, but the principles align with the historical practices and beliefs of the culture, such as spirituality and seeking healing by believing in God. Since the times of slavery, spirituality was a massive part of healing within the Black culture, whether the need is physical or mental.

Black/African American women cope with their mental health by relying on their religious sources while seeking mental health services (Ward et al., 2013). "Similarly, more African Americans (90.4%) than non-Hispanic Whites (66.7%) reported the use of religious coping in dealing with mental health issues" (Ward et al., 2013, Background section, para.6). Researchers believe that for clinicians to see continued success with their Black/African American clients, they should incorporate all social supports, including religion, family, friends, and cultural norms, within the treatment plans for their clients in the communities they serve (Hatcher et al., 2016).

Research Questions

The purpose of this research was to explore mental health issues within the Black/African American community and how African American male and female therapists can grow the utilization of mental health services within the communities they serve. The problem being studied is how the community of Black/African American mental health professionals can breach the topic of mental health with generations of different socioeconomic statuses to bridge the gap between the lack of receiving services and becoming aware of one's mental health status to break generational barriers as well as illnesses amongst the black families in society. The following four research questions will be used to guide this study:

1. What barriers or experiences did potential Black/African American clients think kept them from seeking or receiving mental health services?

2. What practices did potential clients perceive would best fit the Black/African American community's engagement with mental health services?

3. What challenges had Black/African American mental health professionals experienced, working with Black/African American clients?

4. What best practices had Black/African American mental health professionals see that produced the most success in engaging clients or future clients of the Black/African American community?

Description of Terms

Afrocentricity. A line of thinking recognizes the similarities among various ethnic groups but likewise notes that cultural differences should not be ignored, as these variations are crucial to understanding behavior and establishing social unity (Hatcher et al., 2014).

African-Centered Philosophy. A system based on holistic values and ways of living counters the pathological approach that many mainstream workers chose to utilize when dealing with African Americans and other groups of color and insists on practice that honors cultural uniqueness, personal strengths, and community development (Hatcher et al., 2014).

Cultural Competency. The capacity of practitioners and health services to respond appropriately and effectively to patients' cultural backgrounds, identities, and concerns have proposed as a strategy to respond to this diversity and reduce mental health disparities (Kirmayer, 2012).

Discrimination - Occurs when individuals are treated unjustly because of their identities (e.g., race, ethnicity, age, gender). (Hope et al., 2017).

Eurocentrism. A perception in which European (white) values, customs, traditions, and behaviors are used as the exclusive normative standards of merit against which other races and events in the world are viewed (Awosan et al., 2011).

Mental Health Stigma. A set of negative attitudes toward people with a psychological disorder, such as being unpredictable or hopeless in recovery (Masuda et al., 2012).

Phenomenology. A methodological approach that offers access to subjective human experience from the perspective of those who experience it (Ofonedu et al., 2012).

Phenomenology theory. Distinguishes between the various physiological and biological causalities that structure bodily existence and the meanings that embodied existence assumes in the context of lived experience (Davis & Maldonado, 2015).

Contribution of the Study

The Black/African American culture benefits from this study due to the willingness of Black/African American Female and Male mental health professionals to advocate for mental health services and shed light on their journey of working as therapists in the community. Potential Black/African American clients gave their thoughts and opinions of what mental health is, the skepticism behind mental health and seeking treatment, and providing Black/African American therapists with ways to engage the community in seeking mental health services. This research aimed to explore mental health issues within the Black/African American community and how representation of Black/African American mental health professionals can help improve the utilization of mental health services within the communities they serve.

The Black/African American culture in the earlier years steered away from the terminology of psychotherapy or mental health in which has which today more have come around to the idea of seeking mental health services (Williams, 2011). "Mental illness is a health condition that should be of importance in the area of cultural diversity and inclusion because no one is exempt from mental illness, regardless of nationality, race, ethnicity, gender, sexual orientation, or age" (Ward & Besson, 2012, p.2). Mental health seems to have a negative connotation, and due to the barriers and cultural stressors faced, the African American community underutilizes mental health services (Smith, 2015).

Black/African American therapists have addressed challenges faced within their profession and working with the African American community. The challenges stem from a lack of knowledge of mental health, the stigma behind mental health, and the lost progress of their clients due to early withdrawal from the therapeutic process (Williams, 2011). Mental illness has not been an open topic of conversation throughout the Black/African American culture in the past due to the stigma behind it, and many are unaware as well as uneducated about mental illnesses (Williams, 2011). Stigmatization of mental health does not just affect the person diagnosed with it, but it can also affect people associated with them, such as their families (Tew et al., 2011).

For the African American community to be more engaged and seek mental health services, the key, as researchers have gained, is to have more representation of African American female and male therapists (Taylor& Kuo, 2018). With more representation of African American men and women in the mental health profession, it can eliminate the skepticism of feeling misjudged because racially, the client and therapist both connect, which creates a safe environment for one to open and express themselves in a way that they would not with clinicians of the opposite race (Williams, 2011; Hatcher et al., 2016). Potential Black/African American clients perceive that there will not be a lack of cultural competency with an African American clinician due to their shared uniqueness of culture. The connection enhances the client-centered treatment in which the result is progressing with the client (Williams, 2011).

Researchers have noted that mental health stigma has affected the way Black/African American clients view mental health services and because of this, mental health services are not frequently used (Masuda et al., 2012). Black/African American mental health professionals realize that using the Eurocentric theory demeans and diminishes the culture of Black/African Americans, which is not valid and is inappropriate. Implementing the Afrocentric theory in which notes that cultural differences exist among many ethic groups though there are some similarities are essential to understanding the behaviors and perspectives of the Black/African American culture (Hatcher et al., 2016,).

Process to Accomplish

According to Christens (2012), "Psychological empowerment has been theorized according to a human ecological perspective" (p. 542). This theory encompasses the psychological, organizational, and community levels that increase human development (Christens, 2012). A part of human development is taking charge of one's mental health to adapt and adjust, which promotes the resilience of those experiencing mental health issues (Christens, 2012). This study was completed to gain insight into the underutilization of mental health services within the Black/African American community and how Black/African American clinicians can engage clientele.

Research Design

This qualitative research study was designed to encourage and empower the Black/African American community to become more educated on mental health and increase the utilization of mental health services within the community. Qualitative research collects and analyzes data to gain different perspectives and commonalities of a phenomenon (Mills & Gay, 2016). Through this research study, a phenomenological methodology is explored by analyzing common themes and experiences and non-recurring themes throughout the study (Ofonedu, Percy, Harris-Britt, Belcher 2012).

Wertz (2005) described phenomenology as "allowing individuals experiencing a phenomenon to describe their experience exactly as it appears in their consciousness" (Ofonedu et al., 2012, Method section, para. 1). Using the phenomenological methodology approach was appropriate during this research study because each participant expressed through either an interview or focus group their experience on the topic of mental health within the community. The participants were able to voice their concerns, preconceptions, misconceptions, and experiences without restriction, and it gave their experiences a voice (Ofonedu et al., 2012).

This particular methodology was used in a qualitative research study in 2012 to understand the topic of "how inner-city African American youth describe their experience of living with depression" (Ofonedu et al., 2012, The Research Topic Section, para. 1). The research question proposed during this study presented the researchers the opportunity to understand the participants' thought-provoking feelings and experience of living with depression through one-on-one interviews). Giorgi and Giorgi's (2003) phenomenological method approach guided the data analysis by the following steps: (1) Getting a Sense of the Whole, (2) Identifying Meaning Units and Themes, (3) Structural Descriptions, and (4) Composite Description or Essence of the Experience (Ofonedu et al., 2012). By following these steps, the interviews were transcribed to point out meaning units and essential structures to analyze each participant's experience, resulting in the commonality of specific themes (Ofonedu et al., 2012).

The goal of this qualitative research was to explore the careers of Black/African American Male and Female mental health professionals and best practices towards breaking the skepticism towards mental health by answering the four research questions:

1. What barriers or experiences did potential Black/African American clients think kept them from seeking or receiving mental health services?

2. What practices did potential clients perceive would best fit the Black/African American community's engagement with mental health services?

3. What challenges had Black/African American mental health professionals experienced, working with Black/African American clients?

4. What best practices had Black/African American mental health professionals see that produced the most success in engaging clients or future clients of the Black/African American community?

Participants

In this qualitative study, 6-10 Black/African American female and male therapists were invited to discuss socioeconomic backgrounds, educational backgrounds, barriers faced, obstacles they overcame, and what race and culture play in the role of mental health in the community. The researcher wanted to explore how to increase the utilization of mental health services within the Black/African American community and gain insight from the mental health professionals on how they can eradicate the stigma of mental health services within the community.

The participants were identified through networking in the community through different private practices, mental health agencies, and training. The researcher posted an informational flyer regarding the study and those interested were able to reach out via email to the researcher. Once the initial contact was made, consent forms were emailed to each participant. Once the consent forms were completed and returned, the researcher sent out a basic demographics form through email that highlighted each participant's name, age, field of study, credentials, college/university, and place of employment. The participants consisted of Black/African American male and female therapists from different backgrounds regarding education and licensures. The backgrounds of the mental health professionals range from Licensed Clinical Social Workers (LCSW), Licensed Master Social Workers (LMSW), Licensed Professional Counselors (LPC), and Licensed Marriage and Family Therapists (LMFT). Each participant attended a different university and came from different family dynamics as well as backgrounds.

This qualitative study also consisted of 6-12 community participants who were interested in mental health services but were skeptical due to not knowing the first initial steps of seeking therapy and lack of knowledge around mental health services. The researcher put informational flyers of the research study on professional social media network groups and sent the flyer to professional contacts via email. Those interested were able to send an email to the researcher expressing their interest in the research study. Once those participants were selected, they received a consent form, which explained the research study and asked for their signature to participate. After the consent form was signed and returned, each participant received a demographics sheet. Once returned via email or in person, the research study began.

Instruments

The researcher used two different data collection procedures during this research study. The Qualitative research study design consisted of questionnaires that asked about the participants' knowledge, perspectives, or experiences of mental health. The Qualitative research study design also consisted of personal interviews and a focus group. The two methods both used open-ended questioning techniques with probing responses to gather information from the study participants (Guest, Namey, Taylor, Eley, and McKennab, 2017). The investigated areas consisted of what were the barriers of potential clients, Black/African Americans' perception of therapists in the field, influence, and impact of Black/African Americans in the field of mental health, and the retention of mental health in the Black/African American community.

The designed questionnaire instrument was used in a prior study to discuss mental health amongst Black/African American men. According to researchers, there was limited research regarding Black/African American men and their belief system about mental illness; therefore, it allowed more mobility in developing questions for the structured interview (Ward & Besson, 2012). During this study, the exploratory phenomenological qualitative approach allowed the participants to share their thoughts by answering open-ended questions and placed the participants on an equal playing field with the researchers to create a safe space for them. (Ward & Besson, 2012).

Another component of this current qualitative study is collecting data through a focus group with the mental health professionals. According to Guest et al., (2017), "Some scholars assert that the interpersonal and interactive nature of focus groups allows them to produce information that might not be gathered from a single respondent" (p.693). Focus groups typically range from 6 to 12 participants, and the discussion forms as the group navigate through the questions that guide the group (Guest et al., 2017). In this study composed by Guest and fellow researchers, they compared the two instruments of interviews and focused groups on understanding what help-seeking behaviors look like for African American men. Their focus groups consisted of 8 participants, and they used the same interview questions to guide the focus groups as they did the individual interviews. The focus groups consisted of an experienced data collector and an assistant who is typical practice when conducting focus groups. After the focus groups were completed, the data that was collected was audio-recorded and transcribed thoroughly verbatim of what was said from each participant (Guest et al., 2017).

Data Collection

The qualitative study using the phenomenological method approach was completed in two phases. The order of the interviews depended on the date and time of the participants sending back the consent form that was sent via email. The interviews were held and recorded for 45 minutes to an hour, in the fall/winter of 2020 and Spring/Summer of 2021. The researcher obtained consent from the participants to share some of the responses anonymously, although, at the end of the study.

To collect the data to answer research question 1, the researcher identified the seven community participants for the one-on-one interviews. Those interviews took place via video/audio conference. The purpose of the one-on-one interview for the interested participant was to learn about their thoughts, skepticism, and opinions of mental health and how it affects the Black/African American community. The designed interview questions went as follows:

1. What does having a mental health wellness mean to you?
2. What does the term mental illness mean to you?
3. What do you think are causes of mental health?
4. Does the term mental health carry a stigma within the Black/African American culture? If so, why?

5. When thinking of the term, mental health, what are four words that come to your mind? Why did you choose those words?

6. Has mental health wellness been a topic of discussion within your family? If so, can you describe how your family views mental health wellness?

7. Do you discuss mental health wellness with your friends? What are their thoughts regarding seeking mental health services?

8. Describe your image of a therapist?

9. Does race matter when seeking a mental health professional such as a therapist? If so, why?

10. Does gender matter when seeking a mental health professional such as a therapist? If so, why?

11. Is there enough representation of Black/African American men and women within the mental health field?

12. Is mental health discussed enough within the Black/African American culture?

13. Are services underutilized due to lack of accessibility or lack of education of mental health in your community?

14. What do you think are some signs that suggest a person is experiencing a mental illness?

15. How do you feel when you see someone with a mental illness?

16. What do you think can help people with mental illness? Do you think seeking treatment such as psychotherapy or counseling could be a part of treatment?

17. Do you think being diagnosed with a mental illness affects your ability to socialize with others or be accepted within your community?
18. If there is an opportunity to gain more knowledge about mental health, the different diagnosis, treatment, and resources, as well as how it affects the Black/African American community, would you be interested in attending or gaining that information?
19. Advocacy is vital to raising awareness of mental health, therefore, what do you think is needed to continue increasing the awareness of mental health within your community? Would you become an advocate for mental health awareness? If so, how would you raise awareness within your community?

After the interview, the conductor of the interview gave the participant 10-15 minutes to ask questions or reflect upon the interview.

To collect the data to answer research question 2, the researcher used the same questionnaire and received responses from the individual interviews with the community participants to gain insight into what mental health looks like within the Black/African American community. This was essential to gain insight from a personal perspective to generate ideas to propose to the mental health professionals after the research study was completed seeing as these responses are coming from those within the community.

To answer research question 3, the researcher identified the eight mental health professionals who would participate in the one-on-one interviews and the focus group. These interviews would take place via video/audio conference or face to face. The purpose of the individual interview for the mental health professionals was to obtain information about their profession and experience as a Black/African American female or male mental health professional within the community. The researcher conducted a focus group with the mental health professionals to discuss their experiences working with Black/African American clients, mental health disparities within the Black/African American communities, and the influence, impact, and retention of therapeutic services. This focus group took place via video/audio conference. The designed interview questions to guide this portion of the study are as follows:

1. What is your educational background and title? What area of practice do you specialize in?
2. What led you to work within this field and how many years have you been in practice?
3. What does mental health wellness mean to you?
4. In the past, seeking mental health services was looked at as taboo within the Black/African American culture. Do you think mental health is discussed enough within the community If not, why?
5. How has mental health and seeking therapy changed or shifted within the Black/African American community?
6. Are you an advocate of mental health wellness within your family? What types of conversations do you all have regarding mental health awareness?
7. As a mental health professional, is there enough representation of Black/African American women within the mental health field?
8. Does race and/or ethnicity play a role with clients who are seeking a therapist?
9. Does gender play a role with clients who are seeking a therapist? If so, why?

10. Do you meet new clients who mistrust the mental health system and are opposed to psychotherapy? If so, how do you help to change their preconception of mental health?

11. As a Black/African American mental health professional, how do you advocate for the African American community regarding access to mental health services?

12. If you could give a percentage of Black/African American clients that you have served, what would that percentage look like? What age groups are you seeing?

13. How would you have the conversation with a family member or friend to suggest they may need to seek a therapist? How would you gain buy-in from them?

14. As an African American mental health professional, what has been the most significant personal struggle while working in this field?

15. As a mental health professional, how would you gain buy-in from the community you serve and how will you continue to increase awareness about mental health within the Black/African American community?

The interviews were 45 minutes to an hour and were audio-recorded. After the interviews, each mental health professional was invited to the focus group, which would allow each to have a candid conversation amongst other mental health professionals to discuss their thoughts, opinions, and ideas regarding the questions during the interview (Guest et al., 2017).

To answer research question 4, the researcher used the same questionnaire with the eight mental health professionals. The researcher conducted individual interviews and a focus group with the mental health professionals to discuss their experiences working with Black/African American clients, mental health disparities within the Black/African American communities, and the influence, impact, and retention of therapeutic services. This focus group took place via video/audio conference.

The focus group consisted of the researcher, a licensed clinical social worker as the assistant and mediator, the scribe, and the five mental health professionals. Three out of the eight mental health professionals only completed the individual interviews due to time conflicts. The assistant was present to assist with the focus group's logistics (Guest et al., 2017). The designed interview used during the one-on-one interviews was used to guide this focus group. The same questions were used to receive individual feedback and collective feedback to generate ideas to continue to break the stigma and raise awareness of mental health within the community.

Data Analysis

The researcher used the descriptive phenomenological method to guide the data analysis designed by Giorgi and Giorgi in 2003 (Ofonedu et al., 2012). The interviews and focus groups were analyzed using this method which was comprised of four different steps.

To analyze the data collection for research questions 1-4, the researcher started with step one to get a sense of the whole (Ofonedu et al., 2012). The researcher replayed each audio recording of the interview to develop a transcript that read verbatim the participants' responses. The researcher then continued to step two, which was to identify meaning units in which "are non-repetitive, non-overlapping statements that convey a single idea regarding the research question" (Ofonedu et al., 2012, Data Analysis section, para.3). The meaning units were then given codes in which identified the reoccurring themes throughout each transcript, and the codes were used for the participants' names to remain anonymous throughout the study. The codes were also given psychological terms to recognize the different themes within the participants' responses. The researcher then moved on to step three in which allowed the researcher to view the common themes or uncommon themes as structural descriptions, which led to the fourth step, "a statement of that structure, or essence, of the experiences" (Ofonedu et al., 2012, Data Analysis section, para. 5). Within step four, the researcher created case study summaries from the data to obtain the final results in which were recorded according to the themes that derived from each case summary (Ofonedu et al., 2012).

Conclusion

Mental health has an attached stigma, which has caused some African Americans to steer away from it, but with raising awareness and implementing practices to help the engagement of services, the negative connotation of psychotherapy can be seen in a more positive light (Williams, 2011). This research study was completed to continue to help grow the mental health field in the Black/African American community by providing Black/African American mental health professionals with information and theologies to improve engagement of psychotherapy and usage of mental health services in the Black/African American community, but to also motivate more Black/African American male and females to seek the mental health profession as a career choice. The underrepresentation of Black/African Americans in the profession has an immense effect on the underutilization of mental health services within the Black/African American community (Taylor & Kuo, 2018; Beasley et al., 2015). Mental health, viewed as a holistic avenue to heal, will impact, influence, and improve the mental health of the Black/African American community one step at a time when the appropriate practices are aligned (Hatcher et al., 2016).

Chapter II

REVIEW OF THE LITERATURE

Introduction

Mental health is still considered a significant health disparity within the Black community today. Black/African Americans have not received proper and adequate treatment from mental health providers in the past, although they are considered one of the most vulnerable populations of mental health disparities in the United States (Curtis-Boles, 2017). There have been several challenges and obstacles that the Black/African American community has faced with receiving adequate mental health services due to the lack of racially preferred mental health professionals, lack of access to care, lack of resources, and the financial responsibility of seeking mental health care. Many mental health providers who were not of the Black/African American race in previous research presented cultural bias, lacked cultural competence, and this, as well as other factors, resulted in the underutilization of mental health services within the Black culture. Many have made it known that it is not always affordable and, in some cases, when it is reasonable (covered by insurance), the providers do not look like them, which is another barrier to knock down (Curtis-Boles, 2017). Although the obstacles are still there, mental health advocacy continues to raise awareness and increase services such as psychotherapy. This literature review will discuss what mental health means within the Black community and how the illness goes back to the African descent in which studies document the barriers faced and what strategies mental health professionals can put in place to see mental health improvements within the culture overall.

The following research questions guided the literature review:

1. What barriers or experiences did potential Black/African American clients think kept them from seeking or receiving mental health services?

2. What practices did potential clients perceive would best fit the Black/African American community's engagement with mental health services?

3. What challenges had Black/African American mental health professionals experienced, working with Black/African American clients?

4. What best practices had Black/African American mental health professionals see that produced the most success in engaging clients or future clients of the Black/African American community?

Historical Overview

According to Bhugra, mental health has to do with one's self-worth, contributing to self-esteem and overall well-being (Bhugra, 2013). Bhugra also stated that mental health consists of three major components: social, psychological, and physical, contributing to an individual's holistic health (Bhugra, 2013). Mental health within the Black/African American community, in general, was a scarce topic seeing as mental illness was viewed as a weakness within the culture (Shattell & Brown, 2017). Many have experienced racism, discrimination, and mistreatment within the health care system (Campbell & Winchester, 2020). Due to the discrimination and negative connotation that mental illness leaves, Black/African American men and women do not seek mental health care services as often as Caucasian or Latino men and women. Many African Americans experience depression, anxiety, and hopelessness due to cultural stressors (Shattell & Brown, 2017). Mental health can resonate in childhood and carry over into adulthood if not taken care of beforehand (Bhugra, 2013). Those risk factors include household stress, maternal stress, physical abuse, sexual abuse, child abuse, emotional abuse, financial issues, lack of income or employment, and other stressors. Although this plays a significant role within the Black/African American community, there has been an underutilization of mental health services in which some have sought out care through their primary care doctors who may then refer them out to actual mental health professionals, or they will seek help from their religious counsel and social group. Those risk factors include household stress, maternal stress, physical abuse, sexual abuse, child abuse, emotional abuse, financial issues, lack of income or employment, and other stressors (Bhugra, 2013).

According to the World Health Organization, mental health can also be defined as a state where one can deal with life stressors, cope accordingly, and function well within society (Moore et al., 2016). Statistics show that Black/African Americans are more likely to exude feelings of psychological distress at a twenty percent rate. It was also reported that African Americans experience lower treatment rates but have a higher suffering rate when the illness is present (Moore et al., 2016).

Dating back to the 1700s, the church was considered the safest place to express mental health concerns and seek counsel to cope with the daily issues of life (Campbell & Winchester, 2020). The churches formed during these times helped cultivate and navigate the Civil Rights Movement of the 1960s, established grounds for education, and tackled social issues within the community (Robinson, Jones-Eversley, Moore, Ravenel, &

Adedoyin, 2018). The church was viewed as their healing place and remained that way in this day and time. Due to the culture relying on their faith for spiritual guidance with different problems in their daily walks of life, pastors within the Black community are mediators, mentors, and counselors (Campbell & Winchester, 2020). According to research, the church is one place where one feels safe, secure, and heard (Bryant et al., 2015, p. 424). Further study reveals that different Black/African American churches were hosts for access to healthcare within the rural areas (Bryant et al., 2015).

The mistrust of healthcare has existed since the time of slavery. Research shows that white medical doctors and other medical educators relied on Black patients for research studies and did not treat them as people or hold their lives to a more excellent value (Thomas & Casper, 2019). Going back to the freedom of slavery, which guaranteed that Black people would be treated as human beings and have equal rights in 1863, did not change the biases and mistreatment that continue today within the health care system. Discrimination and racism exist within healthcare in which mental health is considered a health disparity within the Black community. Research has proven that those of the minority in the United States suffer from more health conditions in a greater capacity than their White counterparts, but due to historical events, the history of health for Black people has not always been accounted for nor cared for properly. Reaching back to the days of slavery, health disparities within the Black culture and deaths among them were not documented. Other minorities compared to White counterparts' health history was not recorded until 1985 in the publication of the Heckler report (Thomas & Casper, 2019). The Tuskegee experiment "represents a cautionary tale that continues to resonate with African Americans," which has created the idea that providers look at the Black community as research and not human beings (Walker, 2018, p.10). A report completed by the Institute of Medicine in 2002 shared data of cases of unequal treatment of those of the minority who did not receive health care services, such as when bypass surgery or kidney dialysis were needed compared to their White counterparts (Thomas & Casper, 2019).

Moving forward, the minority populations will grow more significantly, and it is said that their status of health will be the baseline within the nation (Thomas & Casper, 2019). According to W.E.B. Dubois, "race and racism continue to be the color line" which "defines the great challenge of our democracy" (as cited in Thomas & Casper, 2019, p. 1347). The right thing to do is to address cultural and racial biases for all to have equal rights to health care seeing as the Black community continues to grow in the population (Thomas & Casper, 2019). The goal is to provide health care services at the same length as others receive and trust that treatment is equally honored to break through the barriers of mental health advocacy within the Black culture.

Global Mental Health

Global mental health research is practices implemented to better mental health worldwide through providing access to mental health locally, distributing resources for mental health in all areas in different communities, appropriate treatment plans to generate positive treatment outcomes (Bischoff, Springer, & Taylor, 2017). Global mental health is the advocacy of mental health, whether on an international, national, or local level, to address cultural and social circumstances. Worldwide, mental health is a disparity experienced by more than 45 percent of the world's population. There are shortages of mental health professionals in the low-income urban areas of the United

States. After the research is completed, policies and practices of the global cognitive research are formed in which then are provided to the communities to improve local access and services that are efficient to improve mental health care. To determine the scope of the problem regarding global mental health, one has to understand the condition of the problem and how critical of an issue it is for specific cultures and communities to gain access to treatment (Bischoff et al., 2017). Expanding the idea of mental health concerns has been categorized as Global mental health, a global subfield of health (Monteiro, 2015). With mental health disparities being a focal issue within ethnocultural groups in the United States, there has to be a change to help break through the barriers and cultivate mental health services to all races and ethnicities to lessen the disparity (Ellis, 2012).

The Black culture in Canada has experienced similar issues regarding health care and the lack of use of mental health services (Taylor & Kuo, 2020). Canada is very diverse, but racism and discrimination were still a factor in the lives of Black Canadians just as it was with Black Americans due to Canada being a country of the White majority. There was a study completed in which 8,000 plus Ontario residents were surveyed, and it showed that Black Canadians experienced more stressful problems in life and less usage of mental health services than White Canadians. The research examined that the lack of utilization of mental health services stems from actual lack of access to care, mental health stigma, education regarding mental health, and cultural mistrust similar to Black Americans' reasoning of not utilizing mental health services. Previous research also noted that the underrepresentation of Black mental health professionals is a common obstacle for them (Taylor & Kuo, 2018).

According to Atilola (2016), the knowledge of mental health is diverse, and some parts within do not have enough adequate information regarding mental illness and mental disorders (Atilola, 2016). Africa is a "multi-ethnic and multicultural region"; therefore, it "is bound to be a deluge of divergent views in sub-Saharan Africa about a deeply cultural concept like mental ill-health, which do not necessarily reflect 'ignorance'" (Atilola, 2016, p. 31). In 2012, the Ghanaian Parliament enacted the new mental health act, which was developed to outline mental health rights for adults and children (Ame & Mfoafo- M'Carthy, 2016). This act consisted of 2 components to protect the right of those diagnosed with a mental health disorder and protect those vulnerable, women, and the elderly (Ame & Mfoafo-M'Carthy, 2016). Mental illness is an issue worldwide and has a significant impact on the quality of life, development outcomes, and other associations resulting from not dealing with mental health properly (Monteiro, 2015). There are not many psychiatrists or mental health professionals in South Africa, and they rely on doctors or nurses, and occupational therapists for mental health interventions (Vergunst, 2018). For example, "based on some data, the density of psychiatrists in or around the largest city is 3.6 times greater than the density of psychiatrists in the entire country" (Vergunst, 2018, p.2). There are only ten to fifteen qualified mental health professionals in Ghana, including psychiatrists and social workers, but their population supersedes that ratio (Ame & Mfoafo-M'Carthy, 2016). Further research shows that "ethnic minority mental health scholars have argued that ethnically mismatched clinicians may not understand the cultural backgrounds or potential cultural response sets of ethnic minority clients" (Kawaii- Bogue et al., 2017, p. 14).

Mental Illness within the Culture

The quality of health care regarding mental health care in different cultures tends to be associated with their cultural identity (Healey, Stager, Kyler, Dettlaff, & Vergara, 2017). Research notes that mental health refers to one's ability to function cognitively, emotionally, and behaviorally (Bishoff et al., 2017). Mental illness is a term that describes a range of disorders that affect ones' thinking, moods, and behaviors (Monterio, 2015). A mental disorder describes the actual condition clinically assessed and diagnosed by a professional therapist (Monteiro, 2015). Clinicians expressed that there are many reasons why mental health services amongst Black/African Americans, such as racial biases that are on display from providers and the stigma associated with mental health. Cultural competence that healthcare providers lack and insensitivity to the client's background (Curtis-Boles, 2017).

The statistics state that Black/African Americans and White/Caucasians both experience mental health at a similar rate, but due to racial injustices as well as lack of cultural competency, the Black/African American community has experienced being overly diagnosed, misdiagnosed, inappropriately treated, and do not receiving the same attention as those of the White/Caucasian population (Curtis- Boles, 2017). Also, in comparison to those of the White/Caucasian race, Black/African Americans are affected due to barriers such as being overrepresented in socially marginalized groups such as foster care, child welfare systems, and prison, which has created a problem with gaining access to care (Kawaii- Bogue, Williams, & MacNear, 2017)

Mental health issues can range from common illnesses such as depression, anxiety, posttraumatic stress disorder, and anxiety to schizophrenia and bipolar disorder

(Madoshi, 2019). Black/African Americans have a 20 percent chance of experiencing these mental health issues than other races and ethnicities (Madoshi, 2019). As mentioned, mental illness can be diagnosed as different disorders, but one illness that gets misdiagnosed within the Black/African American community is depression (Randle, Spurlock, & Kelley, 2019). Depression affects a significant portion of adults in the United States, at the average being around 19 million people. Regarding the Black/African American community, about 9 to 13 percent are diagnosed with major depressive disorder (Randle et al., 2019).

Within the Black/African American communities, it is reported that a large number reside in low-income areas where there are not many resources such as proper health care or education and knowledge about mental health (Madoshi, 2019). It was reported that those who live "in poverty are three times more likely to experience psychological distress than those in affluent neighborhoods" (Madoshi, 2019, p. 61). Research notes that among non- Hispanic Black and White/Caucasian youth, Blacks/African Americans have a higher average of experiencing depression within 12 months (Kessler et al., 2012).

Stakeholders

The stakeholders in this literature review are the Black family. The Black family consists of the mother, the father, and children. The older generation of the Black family culturally coped with societal problems, with their faith at the forefront (Harris, McKinney, & Fripp, 2019). It was reported in 2018 by the Pew Research Center that 83 percent of Black/African Americans believe in God, and 75 percent hold religion as an essential entity in their lives (Harris et al., 2019). It is also stated that Black/African

American women and Black Caribbean women cope with problems by relying on their religion more than men (Harris et al., 2019).

Older Black/African Americans are often underdiagnosed for mental health, more so depression, which leads to not being treated for the illness (Wittink, Joo, Lewis, & Barg, 2009). In the past, the older generation would not seek help for depression because they felt the onset of depression was from the hard times, they experienced and normal (Woods-Giscombe, Robinson, Carthon, Devane-Johnson, & Corbie-Smith, 2016). In this case, the more seasoned generation believed in their religious faith and spiritual being to give them strength during trials, which has impacted their ability to handle issues with mental health and other health disparities (Wittink et al., 2009). Black men in America face cultural and social stressors that lead to health disparities such as mental health, yet they are the least likely to show help-seeking behaviors (Robinson et al., 2018). Many have not sought out mental health services due to the stereotype that was showing emotions is a signal of being weak, which conflicts with gender norms (Hankerson, Suite, & Bailey, 2015). It was reported that only 14 percent of men received mental health care from a professional, of which 29 percent did not seek any professional help (Hankerson et al., 2015). According to this study, Black/African American men were disproportionately exposed to socioeconomic inequalities more than men from other racial/ethnic groups, which increased their stress levels and led to adverse health outcomes (Hankerson et al., 2015). Black/African American males were studied on a college campus, and the results documented Black/African American males suffer from anxiety disorders more than their White/Caucasian counterparts but tend to deal with their emotional/mental health stress alone and are less likely to show help-seeking behaviors (Walker, 2018). African American women undergo psychological stress due to the experience of oppression, their structural and cultural ideals of family and their position of the family, and gendered racism, which ultimately has been deemed the superwoman complex (Woods-Giscombe et al., 2016).

Mental health has an impact on children and adolescents as well as adults. Unfortunately, at a very young age, children of the Black/African American culture are exposed to negatively perceived ideologies regarding their race, and they carry these thoughts and feelings with them as they grow, which affects their self-esteem and self-identity (Taylor, Guy-Walls, Wilkerson, & Addae, 2019). Within the Black/African American community, many facets contribute to the mental health well-being of the children and adolescents, such as adverse childhood experiences, living in poverty or low-income neighborhoods where gang violence is present, not receiving proper health care, or having access to adequate health care (Glasgow, Gerges, Atkins, Molly, & Casket, 2019). In 2017, it was reported that the poverty rate for Black/African American families with children was considerably higher at (33%) at which compared to the Latinx community (26%) and White counterparts at (26%) (Glasgow et al., 2019). Further research found that children who live in low-income, unorganized neighborhoods were 1.9 times higher in experiencing behavioral problems than children who lived in middle/upper-class neighborhoods (Glassgow et al., 2019). According to a child and youth care forum held in 2017, racial discrimination also impacts the youth's mental health, leading to depression and anxiety (Washington et al., 2017). Canals stated that in most racial and ethnic subgroups of children, symptoms of anxiety and depression in most cases have led to adolescents being diagnosed with depression (Canals, Fernandez-

Ballart, & Marti-Henneberg, 2002). When children are experiencing mental health issues, they have a hard time functioning academically and will, in most cases, underperform (Washington et al., 2017).

Families within the Black culture rely on each other for certain aspects to function, but when the basic needs of the team members are not being met in the physiological realm, their mental health is affected and creates more stressors for the family to work through emotionally (McIntosh & Rima, 2007). When the needs of an individual are met with dysfunction, it only adds stress to the team (Lencioni, 2002; McIntosh & Rima, 2007). The dysfunctions of the team come in the form of barriers, in which Lencioni categorized dysfunction into five categories: Absence of Trust, Fear of Conflict, Lack of Commitment, Avoidance of accountability, and Inattention to results (Lencioni, 2002). When the team is in dysfunction, it can lead to more issues such as of lack of job responsibility in which equates to lack of income, children having behavior issues, mother and father struggling to take care of the family, and other issues that can stem from not taking care of one's mental health needs. Mental health has a more significant impact on the family that places greater emphasis on having access to mental health care and raising awareness of mental health to understand better how the team can be in a better place if help is received.

The Black Family: The Role of Support

Those to the Black culture share similar circumstances in their daily walks of life, and it is essential to understand how certain philosophies, cultural norms, beliefs, and tendencies are associated with their ability to function holistically (Cross, Taylor, & Chatters, 2018). Many have experienced discrimination, racism, and oppression in different forms. There are differences between each culture, but the truth that the culture lives in remains the same, the history of Black people consists of a supportive family structure which has been the glue to how the culture continues to move forward (Cross et al., 2018).

Within the Black/African American community, the focus is on making sure everyone is in a good space physically and emotionally (Cross et al., 2018). The support can be in caring for the family of loved ones, childcare, and helping financially. A study was completed in 2004 in which the results showed that 70 percent reported giving their family members emotional support in some shape or form. Within the Black Caribbean community, it was reported that there are 3 million who reside in the United States and represent 7 percent of the Black population within the United States. Many Black Caribbean cultures immigrated to the United States, leaving different family members behind, therefore with ties to their home country, helping financially and filling in as parents to other family members is a practice within their community (Cross et al., 2018).

The role of family support within both the Black/African American and Black Caribbean families is essential in different areas, and most importantly, when finances, socioeconomic status, childcare are a factor, it can create emotional and psychological stress (Cross et al., 2018). The grandparents, mothers, and fathers set the tone for the children, in which those psychological factors can create issues for them growing up in a world where the Black culture is a minority. The grandmother is viewed as one of the most critical family members within the Black/African American family because they provide the most support. Within the Black Caribbean families, it was reported that their support comes from their family, friends, and even teachers in school and that there is an expectation for the youth to succeed due to the amount of social support they have (Cross et al., 2018).

Research shows that the role of the married Black father within the family is to be engaged and involved (Murray & Hwang, 2020). Furthermore, the study suggested that African American men believed in sharing household duties and were responsible for teaching the children morals and values (Murray & Hwang, 2020). When discussing the role of the Black mother, the image that is portrayed is that Black mothers are super strong and must be to protect their children and families (Elliot & Reid, 2016). Elliot and Reid (2016) correlated the Black mothers' efforts to raise their children and save their children from experiencing specific problems such as living in high poverty areas where high crime rates and systematic racism exist to the super strong Black mother image; simply because Black/African American mothers are nurtures of the family and said stressors fall on them (Elliot & Reid, 2016)

Within the Black Caribbean and African culture, parenting and the family looks different than the Black/African American family (Cross-Barnet & McDonald, 2015). Research has found that children are born in a two-parent home where the parents are married. It was also stated that those within the Black Caribbean and African culture have more children in one household than Black/African American families. Their extended families are considered immediate family members within the Black Caribbean and African cultures, making their support more incredible. Furthermore, the fathers are the head of the household and lead the families as far as implementing structure with the children is concerned. Men are considered the breadwinners in the Black Caribbean and African cultures and hold a father to an excellent standard. Family practices are different, seeing as higher family rates within the Black Caribbean culture are formed outside of the marriage. A study conducted in 2005 showed "44% of fathers rated themselves most positively for financially supporting their children, while only 20% said their most positive fathering contribution was being there for their children" (Cross-Barnet & McDonald, 2015, p. 858). It was reported that the mothers within the Black Caribbean and African cultures typically care for the home and take care of the children. Within Africa, mothers usually tend to the house and the needs of the children (Cross-Barnet & McDonald, 2015).

Religion and the Role it Plays within the Black Culture

As mentioned within the Black community, religion plays a huge role, especially within the older generation (Shellman, Granara, & Rosengarten, 2011). Religion seems to be a significant component to helping families regarding their mental health and is the glue to healing with the culture. In the past, being sad or depressed was a weakness of their faith and not trusting God's ability to fix problems in their lives. The church has helped the Black community in four different areas such as prevention, mental health, primary care, and awareness of health (Shellman et al., 2011).

Within the Black Caribbean culture, religion plays a significant role in providing counsel in an emotional and spiritual realm and supporting families immigrating and transitioning to the United States (Rose, Finigan-carr, & Joe, 2017). Religion also helps cultivate cultural morals and values to help the parents pass them down to the children. Furthermore, faith helps to address coping strategies for adolescents to help them get through stressful and challenging situations that they may experience to keep their mental health afloat, especially when enduring immigration. Research has shown that non-

Hispanic adolescents appeared to have a prevalence of mood disorders and psychological/ behavioral issues in the United States compared to non- Hispanic White adolescents. Within the Black Caribbean culture, 15 percent of adolescents who live in the English-speaking Caribbean countries such as Trinidad and Jamaica have more emotional distress that can also appear as depression (Rose et al., 2017).

In Africa, religion plays a significant role in healing and mental health (Read, 2019). They value traditional healers in which rely on their faith (Read, 2019). Traditional healers in the past and even now are advocates for mental health care and work with the African community to provide resources (Read, 2019). It was said that traditional healers and psychiatrists work together to bring appropriate healing and help in areas lacking mental health services. According to research on the history of mental health in Africa, traditional healing was viewed as psychotherapy within that specific culture. Traditional healing is defined as "long-held practices which perceived mental illness as arising from supernatural or spiritual causes" (Read, 2019, p. 619). This motion was set and agreed upon by the World Health Organization, which advocated for traditional healing within Africa's health systems. The movement expanded into several Sub-Saharan African countries where prayer aid in the treatment gap of mental health (Read, 2019).

As mentioned, religion within the Black/African American community is very intricate to their health and well-being (Hays, 2015). Research has shown that Black/African Americans use religious coping practices more than other racial and ethnic groups. Religious coping involves prayer, worship, reading the Bible, and attending church services. According to research, being involved in one's religion within this community has helped promote healthier lifestyles regarding health, mentally, physically, and spiritually. Research studies have found that those who use religion as a coping mechanism have a lower frequency of experiencing mental health issues (Hays, 2015). Preachers with the Black community are looked to for counsel. Therefore, the spiritual perspective is a significant healing component (Campbell & Winchester, 2020). In the past, Black/African Americans were not given the same treatment within health care or social services, and the church was their way of gaining those resources and services. African Americans lean towards their religion and spirituality to help when problems arise in most cases before seeking professional help in mental and behavioral issues (Campbell & Winchester, 2020).

Barriers Seeking Mental Health

It is essential to understand how the barriers affect the Black culture receiving or accessing mental health care. Research has found that those of the minority have less access to care than White populations (Kawaii-Bogue et al., 2017). Those barriers include the stigma associated with mental health, mistrust, affordability, actual access to care (Kawaii- Bogue et al., 2017).

When addressing the under-utilization of mental health services within the Black/African American community, stigma is one of the significant barriers (Taylor & Kuo, 2020). Stigma can be referred to stereotyping someone into a particular group, discrimination, labeling of another person, and or isolating due to a specific problem, illness, cultural bias, and class (Clement et al., 2015). According to Taylor et al. (2019), "Many African-Americans suffer from identity threat, as they believe the stereotypes and identity contingencies assigned to them by the dominant culture" (p. 216).

Mental health stigma involves discriminating against people who may have a mental illness and are labeled due to being diagnosed with a mental illness (Taylor & Kuo, 2020). Under the umbrella of mental health, stigma falls into public stigma and self-stigma (Taylor & Kuo, 2020). Within the Black/African American community, mental health was rarely discussed due to the negative connotation that mental illness brings (Harris, McKinney, & Fripp, 2019). Research has shown that any indication of a mental illness in the Black community makes others feel they have lost their minds and should be institutionalized, which brings on the fear of being ostracized by the community (Taylor & Kuo, 2020).

Public mental health stigma is the fear of being judged by one's family, friends, and community when diagnosed with a mental illness (Taylor & Kuo, 2020). A study was completed in 2018, and results implied that 83% of Black Canadians did not want to seek mental health services due to being judged by family, peers, and others. It is stated that individuals who have been diagnosed with a mental illness within the Black Community are rejected by members of their community (Taylor & Kuo, 2020).

Self- Stigma is the internal judgment that one places on him or herself while dealing with a mental health issue (Taylor & Kuo, 2020). Self-stigma is also addressed as projecting the views others have on a particular group on oneself, which can lead to shame, isolation, and self-esteem issues (Alvidrez, Snowden, & Kaiser, 2008). Research suggests that the Black community experience self-stigma more than other racial and ethnic groups (Taylor & Kuo, 2020).

Within the Black/African American culture, the ideology is that being Black means to be substantial due to the events that the culture has experienced, and having a mental illness suggests that one is weak; therefore, no one in the community wants to be grouped within that stereotype (Taylor & Kuo, 2020). Another stereotype is that one cannot be vulnerable and let their emotions show. These cultural ideologies and beliefs are passed down from generation to generation, leading to mental health being a negative idea and barrier within the Black community (Taylor & Kuo, 2020).

Due to the cultural competency that different mental health professionals lacked when working with those of other racial backgrounds, those of the Black culture were misdiagnosed due to how the symptoms would show (Kawaii-Bogue et al., 2017). With the misdiagnosing of the mental health illness, improper treatment would result in clients being prescribed medication, institutionalized, and possible inadequate treatment overall. A past study in the 1980s showed that when Black/African Americans came in to see their doctors, their complaints would be minimized and overlooked, presenting cultural biases instead of listening to the actual problem at hand. Some researchers suggested that it can cause various diagnoses. For example, when they show more physical symptoms of depression, if not recognized or documented, misconstruing the symptoms could lead to over diagnosing or misdiagnosing the depression, leading to improper treatment. More research has revealed that other races and ethnicities also respond differently to psychotherapy than the White population (Kawaii-Bogue et al., 2017).

Access to mental health care is considered another barrier within the Black/African American community. The Affordable Care Act has integrated primary care services with cognitive/ behavioral health care services within the past few years. However, the model does not encompass frameworks that are tailored to the needs of the African American community, such as being culturally sensitive and eliminating certain biases (Kawaii-Bogue et al., 2017). The integrated model covers older adults and children concerning symptoms of mental health for specific populations and substance abuse disorders, which are rarely discussed within the Black/African American community. Therefore, it is essential to have providers and mental health professionals who are culturally competent and culturally sensitive to understand the history of the culture and help provide appropriate care to those who may lack knowledge of mental health (Kawaii-Bogue et al., 2017).

Mental health care can also be a financial burden to the individual and the family due to insurance only covering a portion of the service cost (Kawaii-Bogue et al., 2017). Being privy to those of the minority living in low-income underserved areas, it may be harder for them to gain access and receive mental health care geared towards one's specific needs. Also, with living in those underserved areas, those in the Black/African American community tend to have more mental health issues that coincide with the disadvantages of living in those areas. Again, the Affordable Care Act supports mental health being integrated with primary care, but insurance does not cover all costs regarding mental health services. Insurance companies cap the number of mental health psychotherapy sessions; therefore, treatment may not work if the individual cannot cover the cost and copay and cost after insurance has covered the allotted number of sessions (Kawaii-Bogue et al., 2017).

Cultural Competency and Cultural Intelligence

Being culturally sensitive ad culturally competent is the ability to use verbal and non-verbal language and cues to show respect and understanding of another's culture, therefore also handling others with care in a way that acknowledges their cultural norms

(Mitchell-Brown, 2020). If one is not culturally competent, one could dismiss another's feelings causing more harm than good when trying to help someone of a different race or ethnicity (Mitchell-Brown, 2020). Black/African Americans felt that mental health professionals were not culturally sensitive to their needs, which formed a negative perspective around being diagnosed (Kohn-Wood & Hooper, 2014).

Mental health practitioners need to be equipped with strategies that serve the African American population, leading to better treatment and treatment plans for better outcomes (Curtis-Boles, 2017). Furthermore, implementing strategies based upon the culture and people shows the clients that one is looking out for their best interests which will develop trust between the clinician and client, resulting in client retention of mental health services (Curtis-Boles, 2017). Cultural competency is a skill taught to health care professionals and consists of five components: cultural awareness, cultural skill, cultural encounter, cultural knowledge, and cultural desire. There is a challenge for clinicians who have formed biases of other cultures to help clients appropriately; therefore, developing a sense of cultural competency through cultural intelligence will help address those biases to better serve the community (Mitchell-Brown, 2020).

There is a trust within the system that has been broken, which goes back to systematic racism and Black/African Americans being judged and treated differently within health care, which has created a barrier between clients and mental health professionals (Kawaii-Bogue et al., 2017). Black/African Americans felt their human rights were being violated due to being used as a medical study during the Tuskegee experiment (Briggs et al., 2014). The Tuskegee airmen experiment exploited

Black/African Americans by not educating them, not treating them, and taking advantage of their socioeconomic status (Bates & Harris, 2004).

The Tuskegee airmen experiment happened in Macon County, Alabama, in 1932 (Paul & Brookes, 2015). The United States Public Health Service ran a study that consisted of 400 Black/African American men diagnosed with syphilis who were never treated, and 200 men who did not have the illness also participated in the study. They were never told they had syphilis and did not consent to be a part of the research study. The study was only supposed to last for eight months but continued for forty years, and within that time, two treatments were developed and available (Paul & Brookes, 2015). Though the treatments were available, the researchers and medical professionals held off treating the Black/African American men to see if the illness affected them differently than other races (Paul & Brookes, 2015). Different officials and local physicians were aware of the study and supported it (Laws, 2018). The study was published, and the ethics of the study were only questioned once during that time (Laws, 2018). Exploiting the Black/African American race by using people as subjects showed how much the government devalued Black/African Americans by emphasizing which race and ethnicity deserve proper medical treatment (Bates & Harris, 2004). The study was unethical but defended because it was medical research (Paul & Brookes, 2015). With this being the perception, mental health care was not too far behind and created the resistance of Black/African Americans assessing mental health care (Briggs, Banks, & Briggs, 2014).

When advocating for mental health services within the community, it is suggested that therapist who is not of the Black/African American culture practice managing underlying biases, racial differences, and certain beliefs to build a positive rapport with clients (Curtis-Boles, 2017). Research has shown that in the mental health realm, clients experiencing mental health issues sociocultural barriers or treatment preferences are not geared towards them in which one would prefer that to be client specific (Delman, Progovac, Flomenhoft, Delman, & Chambers, 2019). When someone is diagnosed with a severe mental illness, they are sometimes not involved in their treatment plan process, creating a lack of engagement and retention with mental health services (Delman et al., 2019).

There are different theories implemented and practices completed when working with clients seeking mental health services. Some approaches that have been implemented in the past by white/Caucasian therapists or psychologists were of the Eurocentric or Ethnocentric theory, which devalued the Black/African American race (Hatcher et al., 2016). Both approaches support racism, social injustice, and biases against the culture (Dune & Walker, 2018; Hatcher et al., 2016). As mentioned, cultural competency is the idea of eliminating personal preferences, understanding others' cultural perspectives, and not forcing one's thoughts on others (Dune & Walker, 2018). Implementing these two theories would diminish the idea of implementing cultural competency (Dune & Walker, 2018). To build a rapport with clients of the Black/African American culture to help them engage in mental health therapy, implementing theories such as the Afrocentric theory and practices that stem from the culture would increase retention (Curtis-Boles, 2017).

Phenomenological Theory

With mental health being considered a health disparity, it is essential to capture and document the impact of mental health and how it was a scarce topic within the

Black/African American community to being advocated for within the culture. The goal of the phenomenological theory is to explore and dissect one's experience (Picton, Moxham, & Patterson, 2017). The phenomenological context acknowledges one's knowledge by analyzing their cultural background, environmental, and socioeconomic factors (Salmon, 2012). The phenomenological theory is used mainly during research regarding mental health because one can gain knowledge through observing and then analyzing it (Picton et al., 2017). Therefore, by completing the investigation, it will highlight internal and external components to what mental health looks like within the community, how the stigma affects one's ability to feel confident in seeking mental health services and will capture one's experience with working as a mental health professional in a community where it can be deemed an adverse health issue to have (Picton et al., 2017).

Continuous Oppression Impacting Mental Health

External factors can affect mental health. As the Black/African American culture strives to advocate for themselves to seek a better quality of care in all aspects, their mental health is being tampered with due to the police brutality and social injustices faced daily (Alang, McAlpine, McCreedy, & Hardeman, 2017). The killings of Black people are all over the news, social media, and being a witness to the social injustice creates a stressor and places fear into the lives of the Black/African community. When police officers are not being held accountable for unwarranted searches, harassment, and deaths of Black/African American men and women, it conveys that Black Lives do not matter. These are traumatic events that have led to one experiencing anxiety, depression, and posttraumatic stress disorder (Alang et al., 2017).

Furthermore, the Black/African American community strives for equality, goes about their daily lives, and tries to work, but carries such a heavyweight on their shoulders (Alang et al., 2017). Many within the culture feel devalued, unsafe, unheard, and scrutinized, linked to poor health. The oppression continues as racial violence is intensified daily. More people within the Black/African American communities seek mental health more than before due to the stress placed and fear formed from the racial injustice and police brutality (Alang et al., 2017).

According to Taylor et al. (2019), the United Nations adopted the Convention on the Elimination of All Forms of Racial Discrimination. However, the United States of America has not followed suit seeing as police brutality, an effective form of racial violence, today (Taylor, Guy-Walls, Wilkerson, & Addae, 2019). Experiencing and witnessing racism can be very traumatic and challenging for one to cope with, especially if it is a repeated trauma. Often, the trauma is downplayed, but several individuals in the Black/African American community are now seeking therapy because the impact brings on stress, sadness, depression, anxiety, and fear. Mental health professionals and mental health advocates such as therapists and social workers need to aid in the push to eliminate oppression, social injustices, violation of human rights, and racism (Taylor et al., 2019).

Aiding in the push for social justice and equality for all races means implementing social justice competency (Smith, 2015). Social justice competency increases the knowledge of resources and individual rights, acknowledges that oppression is accurate, and helps alleviate the stress by mental health professionals advocating for equal access to resources contributing to better mental health services for all (Smith, 2015). Smith acknowledged that mental health clinicians must be educated and address systemic social issues that require a shift in the way clinicians work with clients of a different race or ethnicity. Further research from the Center for Multicultural Mental Health Research expressed that more research should be done to find what strategies will work best to improve mental health in all aspects. All mental health professionals need to be trained in areas of social injustices and inequalities faced by the Black/African American population to advocate for the culture to receive the adequate mental health care they need (Smith, 2015).

Counselors as Transformational Leaders within the Community

Mental health professionals are change agents as well as advocates. Therefore, their roles are significant in what the world is facing today (Smith, 2015). Within the social work profession, those in this field advocate for social justice and economic equality and work to help elevate those in underserved communities by finding resources to help them when in need (Howard, 2018). Many interventions used within the social work realm combat the oppression, discrimination, and systemic racism that the Black/African American community faces daily. When looking at advocacy for social justice and understanding how to elevate those in the Black/African American community through psychotherapy, many clinical social workers use theories and interventions to help build upon the people's strengths and not diminish the history of experienced oppression. When being a change agent, one has to empower others, and in clinical social work practice, social workers lean towards identifying the positive traits of others such as self-esteem, self-respect, and building upon core values to break barriers regarding retention of mental health services (Howard, 2018). The National Association of Social Workers (NASW) and the Clinical Social Work Association commit to being change agents within social justice to better individuals considered the minority within the United States (Howard, 2018).

There was a study conducted in 2017, and the participants acknowledged that "the lack of Black/African American representation amongst counselors" was a reason for them not attending or seeking professional counseling from a therapist (Harris, McKinney, & Fripp, 2019 p. 178). With under 30 percent of the behavioral health care field professionals being Black/African American, the other 70 percent is of different races and ethnicities (Smith, 2015). With the social injustice, police brutality, and racism still present today, more Black/African Americans who want to seek therapy wish to trust mental health professionals with their issues.

Conclusion

There have been countless mentions of clients of African descent not receiving adequate mental health care services, and it has been a great challenge to overcome. Within the last few years, mental health awareness has grown, and more people are presenting help-seeking behaviors in hopes of accessing mental health services. The Black community has and continues to endure different obstacles daily due to oppression, systemic racism, discrimination, inequality of healthcare services, racial profiling, racial violence, living in low-income areas, and lack of resources in which trauma stems from those obstacles. Mental health services were not considered a form of treatment due to the mistrust of healthcare providers and the stigma behind it. Also, other barriers exist, such as affordable healthcare and access to adequate therapy by culturally competent providers (Kawaii- Bogue, 2017).

Due to racial biases and providers who lacked cultural competency, it created a problem of mistrust not only for mental health care but health care in general (Sullivan et al., 2017). Further studies suggest that representation is a vital part of engaging clients of different races and ethnicities within healthcare systems to build trust and increase the utilization of services (Briggs et al., 2014). It is essential for those providing services to understand what it means not to receive adequate mental health care and express empathy to those of the culture (Kawaii- Bogue, 2017). With exuding compassion, there will be a better chance of building a positive rapport with the client, which can lead to better resources being rendered, appropriate treatment planning to serve the client better, and can create retention of services with the Black community seeking and utilizing mental health services (Kawaii- Bogue, 2017). It is said that the mental health field has identified that there needs to be more diversity to combat the underrepresentation of multicultural backgrounds in health care (Fisher, 2019). The mental health field is growing as there is a need for more people of color to advocate for the needs of others. With the mistrust of providers, the social injustice, and stigma of mental health all being factors as to why people may not seek services, it is essential to implement strategies such as more representation of Black therapists, psychologists, and social workers in the field to push towards the retention of mental health services (Mowbray, Campbell, Kim, & Scott, 2018).

The cultural beliefs are similar in that religion plays a massive part in why Africans, those of the Black Caribbean culture, and African Americans chose not to utilize mental health services in the past. Globally, mental health has held a stigma in which kept all cultures from seeking mental health services. The Afrocentric theory was developed in Africa in which carried over into America. With the cultural values, norms, and customs being similar, though there are cultural differences due to geographical residency, some of the issues and barriers remain the same. The reality is that mental health is a problem that more cultures need to be aware of and receive appropriate treatment. Being more knowledgeable of not only one's culture but others can combat different obstacles by implementing cultural competency and cultural intelligence to create better methods to heal the world, end the stigma, and gain access to care, especially in the field of mental health.

CHAPTER III

THE METHODOLOGY

Introduction

This study investigated the experiences of Black/African American mental health professionals and the challenges they have faced with breaking the stigma of mental health within their own culture to increase the utilization of mental health services. Previous research expressed that some of the barriers were lack of access to care, mental health counsel from a professional was out of the cultural norm due to the stigma behind it, and the mistrust of healthcare providers (Hatcher et al., 2016). This study explored the ideologies behind mental health within the Black/African American community and challenged mental health professionals to change the narrative of what mental health looks like within this community by answering four research questions developed to guide the study:

1. What barriers or experiences did potential Black/African American clients feel kept them from seeking or receiving mental health services?

2. What practices did potential clients perceive would best fit the Black/African American community's engagement with mental health services?

3. What challenges have Black/African American mental health professionals experienced working with Black/African American clients?

4. What best practices did Black/African American mental health professionals see that produced the most success with engaging clients or future clients of the Black/African American community?

Research Design

The researcher completed a qualitative study for participants to give individual insight into their internal experience of mental health within the Black/African American community (Ofonedu et al., 2012). Qualitative research aims to collect, analyze, and explain different perspectives to understand a specific phenomenon (Mills & Gay, 2016). Furthermore, qualitative research allows for different meanings to exist and examines those perspectives from multiple lenses to further the ideology behind a particular phenomenon (Mills & Gay, 2016). The information obtained during such research is not modified to produce a certain result, yet it gives the researcher a deeper look into the different experiences and how it has shaped a particular community's outlook on mental health (Mills & Gay, 2016).

This qualitative study was performed using a phenomenological methodology. The phenomenological method is a qualitative way of analyzing common themes throughout the study by understanding the experiences of others as it appears in one's consciousness (Ofonedu et al., 2012). This method was appropriate to analyze the research study because participants expressed their experiences, challenges, and perspectives on mental health within the Black community through an individual interview or focus group.

Participants

Qualitative research requires researchers to closely interact with the study participants; therefore, the sample size of participants in this type is typically small (Mills & Gay, 2016). The small sample size helped the researcher categorize themes and gain a better perspective to produce appropriate study results (Mills & Gay, 2016). In this qualitative study, there were two sample groups: the mental health professionals and the community members. The sample for the focus group was drawn from different mental health professionals who are of the Black/African American race. These mental health professionals ranged from licensed clinical social workers, licensed counselors, and licensed mental health technicians. There was no limit to the age range of the mental health professionals, but the researcher wanted to recruit professionals who had been in practice for more than two years. The researcher identified the participants by networking with different private mental health practices, mental health agencies, and professional training within the community. Also, to recruit mental health professionals, the researcher posted a flyer within mental health professional social network groups. The researcher also emailed the flier to different contacts in her professional network, which received a better response during the recruiting phase.

The sample for the community members was drawn from the flyer of the study being posted on social media platforms and through different social network groups. The researcher emailed the flier to various contacts throughout her professional network as well. There was an age range for the community participants in which they had to be 21 years of age or older. The participants also had to be of the Black and Brown community.

Those interested were able to send an email to the researcher expressing their interest in the research study. The mental health professionals could attend the individual interviews, focus groups, or both. Three mental health professionals completed the individual interviews, and six mental health professionals completed the focus group. The community members were invited to participate in individual interviews, and there were eight participants total for this portion of the study. Each participant of both sample groups: community members (See Appendix A) and mental health professionals (see Appendix B) received an informed consent form before participating. The researcher collected the informed consent forms before the interviews and focus group. Following the interviews and focus group, all were transcribed by the researcher and then coded to protect the participants and to identify specific themes, concepts, and perspectives.

Within qualitative research, the researcher and the participants engaged closely, allowing them to trust the process, open up and become more vulnerable to express their lived experiences (Mills & Gay, 2016). This led to the deeper context in the data collected through the interview process (Mills & Gay, 2016). Ultimately, this will allow both the community members and mental health professionals within the Black/African American community to raise awareness of mental health by gaining insight from others.

Data Collection

The variables investigated were the correlation between the underutilization of mental health services and the skepticism of psychotherapy within the Black/African American community. Mental health is a health disparity amongst all races and ethnicities, and within the Black/African American community, services were underutilized due to the skepticism of mental health (Ward, Wiltshire, Detry, & Brown, 2013). Those within the Black/African American community feared being misdiagnosed, did not trust the health care system, and felt there was a lack of representation of Black and Brown mental health professionals, which contributed to the skepticism of utilizing services geared towards mental health (Masuda et al., 2012). African Americans accounted for 18.7% of the population that experienced mental health illness in 2007, and the number has increased since (Ward et al., 2013).

The researcher used one instrument to collect the data during this research study. Structured interviews are a set of questions that the researcher asks each participant to gain insight into the topic at hand (Mills & Gay, 2016). These questions tend to be open-ended because it allows the participant to give a detailed response and help the researcher obtain deeper insight as the participant is answering the question. Structured interviews also guide focus groups to gain a shared understanding of the topic that is useful in the study. Focus groups allow individuals to come together in a safe space to express their views, perspectives, experiences, and knowledge to lead to a shared understanding (Mills & Gay, 2016). The researcher modified a questionnaire from a research study previously done regarding mental health amongst Black men. The questionnaire was used with the community participants and the mental health professionals during their interviews and focus groups. Therefore, two different data collection procedures during this research study.

This study was conducted using the interviewing method. Both sample groups were captured and recorded on the Zoom video conference platform. The individual interviews were held and recorded for 45 minutes to an hour. After each interview, the recordings were saved in one file and secured with an encrypted password. The researcher was the only individual who had access to the recordings of the interviews. The demographics form and consent forms were also saved with an encrypted password. The researcher assigned numbers to each participant and a group color to differentiate the different study groups for confidential purposes (Ofonedu et al., 2012). After the study was completed, the researcher filed away the physical copies of the analysis and used a lock to lock the cabinet.

This qualitative research study consisted of a questionnaire centered around one's perspective of mental health, their knowledge of the mental illness, and why specific barriers exist within the Black culture. Both the community members and mental health professionals gave their perspectives during the individual interviews or focus groups. The researcher, the participants, and a licensed clinical master social worker were involved during the interview and focus group process.

The data were collected during the Fall and Winter of 2020, Spring and Summer of 2021. Each participant, whether individual or in the focus group, completed the interviews in a safe and secure place for confidentiality purposes. The order of the interviews depended on the date and time of the participants sending back the informed consent form and demographics form that was sent via email. The data were collected at these particular times depending on the participants' schedules. Before the Covid-19 pandemic, the researcher planned to meet the participants in person to complete the individual interviews and the focus group. The researcher secured office space at the local youth and family development center to host the participants and complete the study. Still, during the pandemic, the youth and family development centers were closed to the public. The researcher found it best for the research study to be virtual and scheduled the individual interviews and focus groups according to the schedule of the participants.

Upon IRB approval, the researcher recruited participants by posting informational flyers regarding the study on social media and within professional networks. Those who wanted to participate in the study could contact the researcher by emailing their interest. The researcher then sent back a demographics form as well as an informed consent form.

Once the researcher received the informed consent from the participants, each participant was emailed individually with dates and times to schedule the interview. After the interview was scheduled, the researcher sent a link that allowed both the participant and the researcher to complete the interview process. The researcher gathered certain demographic information at the beginning of the interview and then asked the participant the questions. Nineteen questions were asked during the interview session with the community member participants. The community member participants' interviews were completed before the mental health professional's interviews and focus group. Sixteen questions were asked during the individual interview sessions and focus group sessions with the mental health professionals. After the interviews were completed, the researcher saved the video/audio records in a file that was secured with password encryption. The researcher transcribed each interview to prepare for the analysis of the data.

As mentioned, the research study was completed as a virtual study due to the Covid-19 Virus that placed the entire world into a pandemic. The virus is very contagious and easily spread amongst others. Before the study took place, the researcher planned for the investigation to take place in person, but with the youth and family centers being closed down and other public offices, the researcher decided it was best to complete the study virtually. This changed the trajectory of the study's completion as well. The individual interviews with the community participants and the focus group had to be rescheduled. There were time conflicts with the mental health professionals for the focus group session, which led to a few mental health professionals completing individual interviews. Due to the pandemic, the utilization of psychotherapy increased within different communities, specifically the Black/African American community. The therapists who initially expressed interest in the study, schedules became over packed daily with new and existing clients due to the effects of the pandemic such as the loss of loved ones to Covid-19, loss of jobs, people experiencing depression, having to quarantine and isolate from others, and the rise of police brutality during the pandemic created anxiety amongst the Black/African American Community. Therefore, the researcher had to reschedule the focus group to capture the experiences of the mental health professionals.

Analytical Methods

This qualitative study used the phenomenological method to analyze the data that answered the four research questions by exploring common themes and how mental health has been perceived within the Black/African American community (Holloway, 2015). The phenomenological method captures one's experience; therefore, the phenomenon derives from the data collected; some of the questions may be modified or added during the study to further explore new insights (Ofonedu et al., 2012).

The phenomenological methodology approach was conducted by following four steps which were: (1) to get a sense of the whole, (2) to identify different meaning units and themes, (3) structural descriptions, and (4) composite description or essence of the experience (Ofonedu et al., 2012, Data Analysis section, para. 1-5). The four steps allowed the researcher to understand the different meanings, categorize concepts, and group commonalities of specific themes (Ofonedu et al., 2012).

Step 1: Getting a Sense of the Whole

The researcher listened to the video recordings of the interviews and transcribed the interviews using the Sonix online platform. The researcher wanted to be accurate in transcribing the interviews to fully grasp the concept and understand every participant's lived experience (Ofonedu et al., 2012). It was important for the researcher to clarify each interview and the focus group to analyze the participants' thoughts and perspectives (Ofonedu et al., 2012).

Step 2: Identifying Meaning Units and Themes First

The researcher was able to identify meaning units within the interviews and focus group. The meaning units are considered common words, themes, and/or phrases that mean the same thing (Ofonedu et al., 2012). The researcher gave each meaning unit a code to categorize each phrase, statement, or common word to easily capture what was being said during the interviews. After coding, the researcher documented the meaning units and categorized them into themes. Finally, the researcher analyzed the themes by researching the themes underlying meaning to understand how they correlated to mental health (Ofonedu et al., 2012).

Step 3: Structural Descriptions Here

The third step of the phenomenological method was to transform the meaning units into core structures by using the concept of contemplative experience as well as the imagination of the researcher to understand the participants' experiences, whether as a community member or mental health professional (Ofonedu et al., 2012). The contemplative experience explored the ideas, wisdom, like-mindedness, and openness of the individuals and participants of the study group. While implementing this concept helped the researcher analyze the data, the researcher had to eliminate personal biases to place herself in the same place as the community members to grasp their experience. Through contemplative dwellings and the research being able to apply her imagination to develop themes from the data collected, the researcher labeled meaning units that remained constant no matter what question was asked, therefore categorized as core structures within the study (Ofonedu et al., 2012).

Step 4: Composite Description or Essence of the Experience

Step 4 consisted of the composite structures of the data collected being analyzed to understand each participant's lived experience of what mental health looks like to them within the Black/African American community (Ofunedo et al., 2012). The invariant core structures remained a highlighted theme which allowed the researcher to identify the composite structures of the experiences. The researcher gained clarity by compiling both the core and composite structures together. She was able to finalize the results of the phenomenon that describes the underutilization of mental health in the Black communities.

After concluding the study, the researcher continued to follow Giorgi's phenomenological model (Ofonedu et al., 2012). Within phenomenological research, the researcher does not resort back to the study participants for additional feedback regarding the study's conclusion. The experiences of the Black culture and how they view mental health have caused a lack of utilization of mental health services due to the skepticism behind it for multiple reasons. Therefore, the phenomenological method produces findings that derive their credibility from the correlation of the underutilization of mental health and the experiences of the participants who are of the Black community. The data found from the interviews will confirm whether further research is needed as the essential structures revealed to show why the skepticism of mental health within the Black community exists (Ofonedu et al., 2012).

Conclusion

This study was conducted to understand why mental health a complex topic has been to embrace within the Black/African American communities, why the underutilization of services exists, and how Black/African American mental health professionals can engage the community to take charge of it their mental health wellness. This chapter explored the research method and design used to answer the four research questions that guided the study. The researcher highlighted critical components of the research design and explained the background of phenomenological methodology. The phenomenological method approach was used to conduct this study because it allowed the participants to advocate for themselves and their community by telling their own stories.

Mental health has an attached stigma to it which has caused some within the Black/African American community to shun away from seeking help (Williams, 2011). Therefore, the researcher captured the perspectives of individuals within the Black/African American community to voice what mental health once looked like and how advocacy amongst the different generations can empower others to engage in the services offered. During this study, mental health professionals of the Black/African American community shed light on the challenges that many Black/African Americans face and how they can affect one's mental stability. Both sample groups acknowledged that as a culture, there were apprehensions around mental health and as time has changed, so has the need for mental health services such as psychotherapy to be utilized. Their personal experiences aligned with previous research during this study, yet it created an avenue for change by exploring culturally historical ideologies and curating opportunities to restore one's outlook on mental health.

Chapter IV

FINDINGS AND CONCLUSIONS

Introduction

Within the Black/African American culture, being diagnosed with a mental health illness or seeking help for mental health created negative and cultural stigmatization (Taylor & Kuo, 2020). Unfortunately, this ideology was passed down from generation to generation, in which cultural stressors and other life struggles have led to depression, anxiety, fear, and anger (Shattell & Brown, 2017). Over the years, different celebrities, athletes, and mental health professionals of the Black/African American culture, such as actress Taraji P. Henson, NFL star Brandon Marshall, and gymnast Simone Biles, have spoken out about the importance of taking charge of one's mental health which has increased the awareness of mental health. The findings of this research will continue to cultivate the idea of mental health being accepted within the Black/African American communities.

This study was conducted to understand why there was an underutilization of mental health services by addressing the barriers presented by previous research as well as confronting some of the issues by speaking with community members and mental health professionals on how to change the perception by answering four research questions developed to guide the study:

1. What barriers or experiences did potential Black/African American clients think kept them from seeking or receiving mental health services?

2. What practices did potential clients perceive would best fit the Black/African American community's engagement with mental health services?

3. What challenges had Black/African American mental health professionals experienced, working with Black/African American clients?

4. What best practices had Black/African American mental health professionals see that produced the most success in engaging clients or future clients of the Black/African American community?

Findings

This chapter will first explore the common themes of the structured individual interviews. The researcher identified meaning units and coded them as different labels. These themes highlighted the lived experiences of each participant as well as their thoughts and perspectives towards the questions that were asked during the structured interviews.

RQ 1: What barriers or experiences did potential Black/African American clients think kept them from seeking or receiving mental health services?

To answer research question one, four themes emerged during the individual interviews with the community participants: stigma, lack of access, lack of education, and racial preference.

Figure 1

Highlighted Themes During Individual Interviews

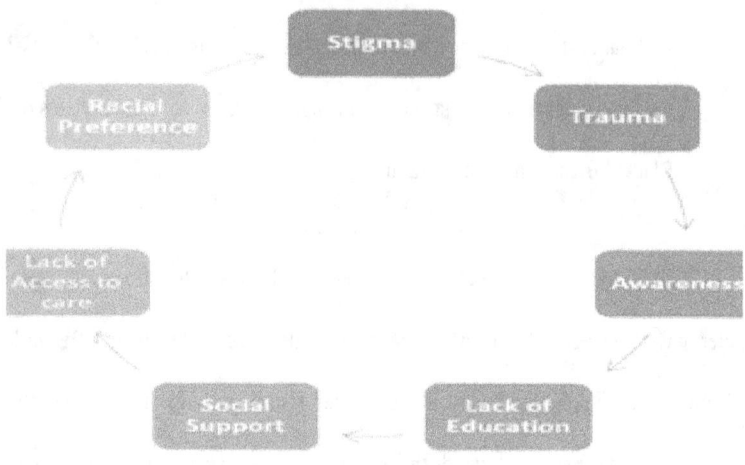

Note. This figure demonstrates the highlighted themes that appeared within each of the individual interviews that the researcher conducted with the community participants.

Stigma

It carries the stigma that you're crazy, something is wrong with you, you need help, and that's the truth, I do need help. (Community Participant 1)

Cultural stigma was expressed as a reason as to why those within the Black/African American community do not seek mental health services. It was said that historically, mental health was associated with someone being crazy or that their mind is not fully functioning, and others found the phrase mental health to be humiliating. It was said in the interview that within the Black culture, problems that arise, such as mental health, are swept under the rug. Ultimately, mental health stigma caused Black/African American families to fear accepting services or even seeking them because they did not want to be labeled as someone with a mental health problem.

> *It's becoming a good thing.* (Community Participant 5)

Although many families have felt that mental health stigma is a barrier, those within the millennial generation have started to embrace that everyone has experienced some form of trauma and wants to combat mental health stigma. Others realized that they must be the ones in their families to break down the barriers by being the first to attend therapy or seek different mental health services. The Silent Generation and Baby Boomers are still working their way through understanding that mental health is just as important as their physical health.

Lack of Access

> *I would like to see events where people take advantage of their resources, such as highlighting different therapists, discussing lowering rates, or taking specific insurances.*
> (Community Participant 4)

Participant 4 felt that therapy could be expensive, especially for people who do not have insurance. When she started feeling specific ways and could not meet with her therapist, she found new ways to add positivity to her life by exploring a hobby and journaling. It was expressed that even though most jobs offer EAP, those only consist of six free sessions. Participants have great hopes that as the utilization of mental health services increases, especially during the pandemic and after, individuals can seek more affordable and accessible therapy for those who want to seek services.

Lack of Education

> *I think the biggest reason mental health is such a rarity in our community is a lack of education. You have this widespread ignorance about you, which is why the negative connotation has been carried from generation to generation.* (Participant 1)

Participants reported that when they were younger, mental health was not a topic of discussion. Now that it is pertinent to survive, the community wants to learn how mental health affects one's overall well-being. One of the participants expressed how when he was a child, he would be labeled by adults because of his behaviors, but no one asked him why he was feeling a certain way or what triggered him, but as an adult, he has done research to understand what trauma is, what mental health looks like when one is not stable, and how he can help others who cannot verbalize what they need to be in a better mental space. It was expressed that those within the Silent generation were not privy to mental health education due to inequalities within healthcare. Furthermore, the disparities of health care and systemic racism contribute to a significant portion of the lack of mental health literacy and the fear of seeking the help needed.

Racial Preference

I think it's super important that whomever you're sitting with is aware of that, that they have that knowledge and that education. I don't think they would be able to serve you beyond the surface if they don't. I've been upset with White counselors because they counsel based on what their textbooks have said. (Community Participant 1)

While speaking with the participants during their interviews, each participant expressed an underrepresentation of Black/African American men and women within the mental health field. One participant said that he did not have a good experience with a clinician of another race, and he felt the clinician could not help him because they could not relate to each other. Another participant explained to the researcher that it is vital that the mental health professional makes the client feel heard and valued; she went a step further to disclose that her therapist understands what it means to be a Black woman in today's world and that she just gets it. Many of the participants preferred their clinician to be Black/African American due to the struggles, cultural stigmas, historical traumas, and the ability to trust someone who will not look down on them because of the color of their skin or because of cultural biases.

RQ 2: What practices did potential clients perceive would best fit the Black/African American community's engagement with mental health services?

To answer research question two, five themes emerged during the individual interviews with the community participants: a safe space to understand trauma, awareness and unmasking emotions, social support, lack of access, and racial preference.

Safe Space to Understand Trauma

If you were raised in a home where there was much violence or much turmoil, much instability, it just ended up shaping you who you were, a lot of us think of that as normalized behavior. (Community Participant 3)

Within the interview, the participants correlated mental health with trauma, and a few of them recognized that their childhood trauma was showing up in adulthood. The participants discussed how trauma could be losing a parent at a young age, seeing their parents argue and fight, or being in survival mode and having adult responsibilities as a child. Furthermore, the participants discussed how their trauma can bleed over into their children's lives and that it was essential for them to deal with the unspoken trauma to be better parents, partners, friends, and colleagues. The participants expressed that those specific triggers have created negative spaces that have led to anxiety, depression, or just a form of sadness that they have not expressed verbally. Some participants have attended psychotherapy to start working through their traumas, whereas others are still trying to figure out if therapy is the right direction to take.

Awareness and Unmasking Emotions

I would get labeled as at-risk or with all these different labels about behavioral challenges and stuff like that. While they were speaking to, I guess, like the byproduct, they were not having a conversation with me about where any of it was stemming from. At age six, I was sitting and living in all these feelings that I didn't have context for, and I didn't have language. (Community Participant 1)

Being aware of one's mental state is essential and knowing how to address specific fears, feelings, and self-doubts are a considerable component of knowing when to seek help. Within the interview, the ability to self-regulate one's emotions when problems arise is a discussion component. There has been this underlying expectation that men and women within the Black culture should mask their feelings to not seem weak around others, and this has been passed down from generation to generation. One of the participants spoke to the issue of Black men not having safe spaces to express themselves, and how ultimately, it has led to sadness, isolation, depression, mental breakdowns, and has also caused families to become broken because of emotional suppression.

Social Support

I realized the importance of having social support and having brothers and sisters that you can talk to and just release. (Community Participant 5)

Within the interview, participants expressed they have a support system and that those supports consist of their friends, younger relatives, and parents. One of the participants felt he has only been able to communicate his struggles with mental health with his siblings and cousins; the conversations with his aunts and uncles have been surface level. Another participant felt as if she could only discuss issues with her friends but realized she needed a mental health professional to sort out her feelings after a drastic life change happened. Many of the participants felt their friends supported their healing journey by seeking mental health services such as psychotherapy.

Lack of access

Counseling is a luxury, and so I think we must introduce the concept of self-healing. I do believe there are ways that we can heal and journey through mental wellness.
(Community Participant 1)

When the participants discussed mental health awareness and what it meant to them, a couple mentioned that when one is aware that they struggle with mental health issues, they can apply the tools they have learned, such as coping mechanisms, to help them along their journey. Participant 1 explored the misconception of psychotherapy as the only technique to help an individual experiencing mental health issues. He suggested that individuals should implement different strategies as well as resources for coping mechanisms. Participant 3 feels people must accept mental health to start the process of seeking a therapist or services.

Racial Preference

It was something different about my fourth-grade teacher. It was something different about my high school counselor. It was something different about all these people; they looked like me, and even though I didn't say it, we all felt the same way. It matters.
(Community Participant 7)

While speaking with the participants during their interviews, each participant expressed that there is not enough representation of Black women and Black men in the mental health field. Through the interviews, the researcher gathered that majority of the participants were raised by generations of men and women who constantly fought the battle of does mental health existed, and it was their job to combat the stigma to break the generational skepticism of it to heal individually, as a family, and as a community. The community participants dove deeper into systematic racism and social injustice and expressed that 2020 was more than a year of clarity, but a realization that healing must take place, and it starts by increasing awareness of mental health. The researcher examined the ages of the participants closely, and each participant was between twenty-eight to forty years old. She felt that seeing more Black women and Black men in the healthcare field and mental health field would have increased the chances of those children growing up to attend college to follow those same career paths. She talked about how her fourth-grade teacher and her high school counselor were Black and that it influenced her to go into those fields because they showed her that they cared.

Mental Health Participants

Next, the researcher identified common themes within the individual interviews and focus groups of the mental health professionals. The researcher identified meaning units and coded them as different labels. These themes highlighted the participants' lived experiences and their thoughts and perspectives towards the questions during the structured interviews. Although the individual interviews and focus groups took place at different times, frequent themes emerged from each participant.

Figure 2

Curated Themes During the Individual Interviews and Focus Group

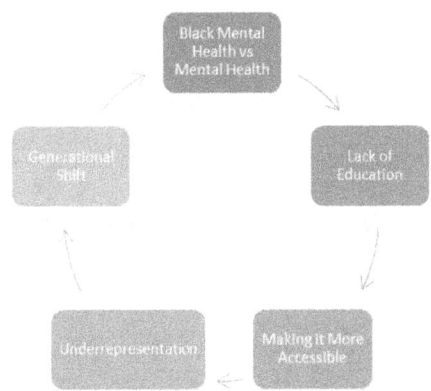

Note. This table demonstrated curated themes identified from the individual interviews and focus group that the researcher conducted with the mental health professionals

RQ3: What challenges had Black/African American mental health professionals experienced, working with Black/African American clients?

To answer research question three, three themes emerged during the individual interviews and focus groups with the mental health professionals: Black mental health and mistrust of healthcare providers, lack of access, lack of education, and racial preference.

Black Mental Health and Distrust of Health Care Providers

My grandparents would have been that silent generation, like their generation, is different, and we can understand why they're different. But with that, you don't talk about anything right, or we mislabel things. And so, many misconceptions and even distrust for medical professionals, which I think mental health would fall up underneath that as well, come from that silent generation. (Participant 6)

> *Black mental health is vastly different because of the number of things that continue to happen in our community that doesn't seem to occur in other societies. I mean, if we look at what happened last year, you know, it was very publicized, the killings of Ahmaud Arbery and George Floyd, and how that affected all of us as people of color.*
> (Participant 1)

Previous research of mental health within the Black culture explored mistrust of healthcare professionals in the past due to different medical studies. Participant 6 expressed how the older generation did not speak on their issues due to distrust. It became more apparent that they remained silent to prevent themselves from being misdiagnosed or taken advantage of by healthcare professionals. Participant 6 expressed that because mental health was not discussed, it did more harm because mental health has always been an ongoing disparity, but the terms such as trauma were not taught; therefore, specific problems were never identified or faced.

Lack of Education

> *I've experienced that generation of women where it was highly taboo to have something wrong with you or be considered crazy. I can remember being young and hearing my mom say, oh, that's so-and-so who had a nervous breakdown.* (Focus Group Participant 3)

> *Psychotherapy provides mental health services for people who are dealing with trauma, maybe grief, have a mental health diagnosis. Which could look like bipolar disorder, depression, anxiety, things like that.* (Participant 8)

The participants within the focus group discussed the lack of literacy behind mental health; some expressed that it was ignorance and the act of not embracing what mental health is. Participant 8 felt that literacy was lacking regarding mental health and psychotherapy. Also, the participants expressed that the community may not quite understand the different diagnoses such as anxiety or depression and how it can affect someone's ability to function daily.

Underrepresentation

There are not enough men in the profession, and then with that, there is an even more so more minor degree of black men. (Focus Group Participant 4)

This is the first time that we've ever hired a black male therapist; so, for me to say that is kind of disheartening because our children need positive role models to look up to who look like them, who are different than what they are typically exposed to or have experienced. (Focus Group Participant 6)

They want a therapist who looks like them because so much of them comes into the therapy room. There's a lot you don't want to have to explain, and there's a lot you don't have to give the back story on. Someone who just gets it is what a lot of Black and Brown clients are looking for. (Participant 6)

The mental health professionals all dove into how the pandemic, racial and social injustices have triggered the Black/African American community. They expressed how they have seen an influx of clients due to individuals not feeling safe, feelings of depression and anxiety, feelings of being unwelcomed, anger towards authority, and many have become aware that they are suffering from past traumas that were triggered by the killings of George Floyd, Breonna Taylor, and the protests that were ongoing throughout the pandemic. Each mental health professional expressed that the word trauma has surfaced multiple times and that the pandemic created a mental health awareness movement or trend that is steadily growing. A few participants said that racial preference allows individuals to be more transparent and vulnerable and feel accepted. The participants addressed how the stigma of mental health is slowly fading away, but with that, it will take more Black and Brown, mental health professionals entering the field to match the increase of clients.

RQ 4: What best practices had Black/African American mental health professionals see that produced the most success in engaging clients or future clients of the Black/African American community?

To answer research question four, three themes emerged during the individual interviews and focused group with the mental health professionals, which were accessibility and generational shift.

Accessibility

The pandemic has done many things, good, bad, and indifferent. I won't go down that road, but I will say that the pandemic has allowed mental health to become more accessible. (Focus Group Participant 1)

Within the focus group, two mental health professionals offered psychotherapy through virtual platforms, just as medical professionals do by providing telehealth. Focus group participants 1 and 2 felt they received an influx of new clients at the breach of the pandemic, and it increased when racial and social injustice were publicized. Participant 8 expressed that she has been able to help individuals through her social media platform and that it has been another way for people to access mental health literacy as well. Within the individual interviews, Participant 7 mentioned that her private practice looks into their workshop training centered around mental health, trauma, grief, male masculinity, and mental health, which is accessible to the community through their YouTube channel. It was mentioned that some agencies offer psychotherapy on a sliding fee scale for individuals who do not have insurance. One participant touched on the Employee assistance program services (EAP) that most jobs offer to employees, which allows for six free counseling sessions.

Generational Shift

The literacy part of it is just really understanding what trauma is and understanding what oppression has done and not just pressure before, but also like the oppression of where we are now. (Focus Group Participant 1)

One of the things that I think could potentially be helpful is seeing the number of athletes speaking out towards mental health, especially those of color. A generational shift of where we are is also helping more people become more comfortable with seeking out mental health services. (Focus Group Participant 4)

In both the individual interviews and focus groups, mental health is more accepted within the Black/African American community and has been going in a more positive direction over the last few years. The mental health professionals attribute the growth to mental health being a topic of discussion on a more public platform such as social media. It was expressed that many individuals follow the trend promoted on social media and that "mental health" has become a buzzword (Focus Group Participant 1).

I work with many families to see the teenager and mom separately, then I might see them together. (Participant 7)

A few participants discussed how an individual's mental health could be affected by their environment, vice versa, and sometimes family therapy is needed. With the generational shift, the mental health professionals mentioned that the millennial generation had embraced the idea that mental health is a part of being healthy overall, and with that, they have empowered generations before them to seek therapy. One of the therapists expressed that it is hard to heal in a broken environment, and in many cases, that is what the mental professionals see when working within the Black/African American community.

Summary of Findings

Through the interviews with both sample groups, the researcher depicted several commonalities throughout the study. The researcher gathered that most of the participants were raised by generations of men and women who may have constantly fought the battle of whether mental health exists and did not want to be labeled as another statistic. The researcher examined the ages of the participants closely, and each participant was between twenty-eight to sixty years of age. Each participant expressed that either themselves, a family member, or a friend has experienced struggles with mental health and would like to be more knowledgeable on how to receive services such as psychotherapy. The lack of mental health literacy has prohibited a lot of healing within the Black/African American communities. This study has opened another gateway for linkage to care and has raised awareness of mental health by understanding the experiences of the individuals within the study. Whether the individual was in the community sample group or the mental health professionals sample group, each participant highlighted that past cultural norms, past and present traumas, and the stigmatization of mental health led to the underutilization of service. Many mental health professionals have worked hard to change the narrative within their respected organizations, agencies, and communities. The significance of the phenomenology behind mental health is that both sample groups are change agents for their families, friends, communities, and clients served by combatting the stigma and breaking the generational skepticism psychotherapy as a treatment method.

Limitations

The researcher encountered different limitations while conducting the study. The first limitation was gaining the participants. Mental health is such a broad topic but requires in-depth conversations. Knowing that it is a scarce topic within the Black culture, the researcher predicted that there would be some hesitancy with community members wanting to participate. The researcher promoted the study for almost three weeks before receiving inquiries from individuals wishing to participate in the study. Due to the study being a qualitative design, the researcher could use the small sample size she obtained to conduct the study. Regarding the mental health professionals and licensed clinicians, the researcher did not have a hard time gaining participants, but there were conflicts in schedules due to the nature of the work.

Second, Covid-19 created different problems for the researcher, with the first challenge being the study changing from in-person research to a virtual analysis. The researcher planned to use one of the local youth and family development centers to host the study. It was essential to the researcher that she picked a place that was central to the participants. The researcher also selected a unique location as it was one of the youth and family development centers that remodeled to bring a new sense of hope to the community. Unfortunately, Covid-19 affected the community facilities, and the youth and family development centers were closed to the public. The researcher wanted to ensure everyone stayed safe and healthy during this time.

The third limitation was time constraints. The pandemic caused individuals within the healthcare field, including mental health clinicians, to be considered frontline workers or essential workers. Due to this, some clinicians saw an influx of clients, which created a time barrier for the focus group. The researcher rescheduled the focus group a few times on behalf of the mental health professionals and herself as she was also considered an essential worker. After the individual community participants' interviews were completed, the therapist worked around the mental health professionals' schedules to complete the focus group. Three mental health professionals could not participate in the focus group, but they completed individual interviews because they still wanted to be a part of the study.

The last limitation was, of course, technology. During some virtual interviews, the screen would become frozen, or the signal would fade, but both the researcher and participants worked through it. The pandemic was a part of history that no one could predict. Therefore, the researcher continued to work through the issues by communicating with the participants and working around their schedules to complete the study.

Implications and Recommendations

The researcher gained a new perspective about mental health and mental health professionals work within the community. Mental health professionals consist of clinicians, social workers, licensed professional counselors, psychologists, psychiatrists, mental health technicians, and behavior specialists. The researcher's educational background is that of the social work field, and she has done the work within the area as a mental health advocate and clinical clinician. During the study, learning from other mental health professionals allowed the researcher to see how the practice has changed within the last three years from mental health professionals who have been in practice for over eight-plus years. It was important for the researcher to learn more about the barriers and challenges that the mental health professionals experience and work through daily, primarily because few Black/African Americans work within the mental health field. The messaging in the past was that Black/African Americans should not go into the mental health profession, again stemming from the Silent Generation and Baby boomers experienced in the past with inequalities in healthcare. It is estimated in 2012 that only 27.9% of Black/African Americans were represented in the mental health professions in the United States (Smith, 2015). Over the years, that number has changed, and the domain is growing. Still, after speaking with the community participants, in which the majority were in the southeastern part of Tennessee, they expressed that there is still a lack of Black/African American clinicians.

Furthermore, by interviewing the community participants, the researcher was able to see a refreshed mindset of mental health being accepted. It was reported that Black/African Americans were more than likely to show feelings of psychological distress but had lower rates of gaining treatment (Afalava, 2020). Most of the community participants expressed that if their parents or grandparents were to participate in this study, the conversation would have been a lot different, as most of the participants come from the Baby boomers or Generation X while their parents and grandparents came from the Silent generation. Unfortunately, those within the millennial and generation z age groups must unlearn the silent patterns and address mental health by getting through those barriers. The researcher learned that more community members want to know how mental health affects their overall well-being, and they want to change the narrative by setting the example that mental health is just as important as one's physical health. For so long, mental health has carried a negative connotation. Through this study, the researcher was able to gain information to help advocate on behalf of those within the Black/African American community searching for resources.

Due to the limitations of the sample size, the researcher would recommend that this study be duplicated in different geographical areas. One of the study participants lives in Atlanta, Georgia. He expressed that it is not hard to find a Black/African American therapist in his area but that Black/African American clinicians are still underrepresented statewide. It would be interesting to see the different perspectives of mental health professionals and their experiences from other geographical areas.

Another recommendation would be to complete the study in person. With the pandemic taking place, the researcher had to opt to complete the study virtually. The researcher experienced very transparent moments with all participants of the research but feels there would have been more participation for the focus group if there was an in-person setting. Ultimately, the researcher wanted to run two focus groups with the community members and mental health professionals but did not receive enough participation.

Lastly, the researcher recommends that the researcher reaches out to different organizations, churches within the community, Black/African American owned private practices, as well as other mental health agencies to gain insight from individuals who are of the Silent Generation, the baby boomers, Generation X, Millennials, and Generation Z. This would have sparked different conversations and gave more insight to the historical perspective of what Black Mental health looked like years ago. This would provide more substantial research into how the narrative of mental health has changed within the Black culture.

Conclusion

The Black/African American community has struggled and endured intrusive obstacles such as systemic racism, racial and social injustice, inequality of health care, and other life stressors that have caused different traumas to form. Seeking mental health services such as psychotherapy was not considered a form of treatment for years due to cultural beliefs (Kawaii- Bogue, 2017). Furthermore, the utilization of mental health services was used at a lower rate for those of the Black/African American race due to mistrust of the healthcare system, lack of resources, the stigmatization that comes from being diagnosed with a mental health illness, and there being an underrepresentation of Black/African mental health professionals (Kawaii- Bogue, 2017).

This research study was conducted to further the exploration of the phenomenology of mental health. By gaining insight from the Black/African American community and Black/African American mental health professionals, the researcher's goal was to merge the two components to change the narrative of mental health and increase utilization within the culture. The underrepresentation of Black/African Americans professionals in the mental health field has a vast effect on the underutilization of mental health services within the African American community;

therefore, the researcher also hoped to encourage those within the field to continue the groundwork and advocacy to build upon the resources that are accessible to those within the community Black/African American individuals to support the movement of raising awareness of mental health by (Taylor & Kuo, 2018; Beasley et al., 2015).

  The researcher cultivated the phenomenology of mental health after analyzing the data collected from the study. The themes derived from the study gave the researcher a greater perspective of what mental health looks like within the Black/African American community. Through extensive research and structured interviews, the result of the study was that the community participants and mental health professionals both had experienced some of the same issues with the acceptance of mental health. Both sample groups acknowledged that it had been a slow process to get the Black/African American community on board with the understanding that mental health is a health disparity and should be taken care of just as one's physical health should be. The researcher learned from the community participants that safe spaces are needed to combat the stigma of mental health due to generational traumas and cultural norms, and it can be not easy to gain support from others when seeking help. This study gave both sample groups a voice to raise awareness of mental health by speaking on their individual experiences to change the narrative. The researcher created a resource directory guide for the community to direct them to mental health services and shed light on how the skepticism has decreased due to the generations speaking up and taking charge of their overall well-being.

www.ingramcontent.com/pod-product-compliance
Lightning Source LLC
LaVergne TN
LVHW020425080526
838202LV00055B/5044